Obesity Surgery

University of Nevada Press
Reno & Las Vegas

Marta Meana Ph.D. and Lindsey Ricciardi Ph.D.

Obesity SURGERY

Stories of Altered Lives

University of Nevada Press, Reno, Nevada 89557 USA
Copyright © 2008 by University of Nevada Press
Manufactured in the United States of America
Design by Louise OFarrell

Library of Congress Cataloging-in-Publication Data
Meana, Marta, 1957–
Obesity surgery : stories of altered lives / Marta Meana and
Lindsey Ricciardi.
   p. ; cm.
Includes bibliographical references and index.
ISBN 978-0-87417-739-8 (hardcover : alk. paper)
ISBN 978-0-87417-740-4 (pbk. : alk. paper)
1. Obesity—Surgery—Patients—Interviews. I. Ricciardi,
Lindsey, 1976– II. Title.
[DNLM: 1. Bariatric Surgery—psychology—Interview.
2. Obesity, Morbid—psychology—Interview. 3. Obesity,
Morbid—surgery—Interview. 4. Weight Loss—Interview.
WD 210 M4830 2008]
RD540.M432 2008
617.4'3—dc22   2007048452

The paper used in this book is a recycled stock made from
30 percent post–consumer waste materials and meets the
requirements of American National Standard for Information
Sciences—Permanence of Paper for Printed Library Materials,
ANSI/NISO Z39.48-1992 (R2002). Binding materials were
selected for strength and durability.

First Printing
17 16 15 14 13 12 11 10 09 08   5 4 3 2 1

This book is dedicated to the gracious women and men in these pages who gave so generously of their life, time, and stories so that others could benefit from their experience.

Contents

Preface

This book has no agenda other than to provide the reader with a collective account of life before and after obesity surgery from the perspective of a group of individuals who are likely to be representative of many people opting for this surgery. This is neither a pro- nor an anti–obesity surgery book. It aims simply, or perhaps complicatedly, to explore how this procedure can affect lives. As a matter of fact, every one of the individuals we interviewed, regardless of all manner of postsurgical dilemmas, told us they would have the surgery all over again in a heartbeat. But almost all of the people we interviewed also said that they were completely unprepared and flabbergasted at the psychological and social upheaval of losing that much weight so quickly. This was true even when the changes were long wished for. That is the focus of this book. We simply wanted to know what happens to the psychological and social lives of people who step out of clinically severe obesity.

Part I consists of five chapters organized around the interviews we conducted and the stories our interviewees told us about life before and after the surgery. These chapters cover the motivations for surgery and then the changes that the weight loss caused in relationships and in their self-concept. Part II consists of two chapters: One summarizes our interviewees' experiences into a model of the postsurgical process and delineates the path that most of their experiences appeared to follow. The last chapter presents a step-by-step program to help individuals who are considering surgery, or who have already had it, prepare for and cope with the changes they will experience. We hope that this account of pre- and postsurgical life and our recommendations will accomplish the following:

1 contribute constructively to deliberations about whether or not to have the surgery

2 help prepare and equip individuals who are either waiting for or have just undergone weight loss surgery

3 validate the experience of those who have gone through it

4 inform the interventions of health care professionals who treat and support individuals through this process

5 help partners, relatives, and friends understand and support the psychological journey their loved one is undertaking.

In addition to the men and women who shared their stories with us, we are indebted to a number of other important people and one institution in the writing of this book. First and foremost, we would like to thank Dr. Barry Fisher for giving us entry into the world of his patients and for sharing his insights. This research project would have been impossible without him. Dr. Chris Heavey, our dear friend and valued colleague at the Psychology Department, University of Nevada–Las Vegas, convinced us that this story needed to be told more widely. This research project might never have become a book without his insistence. The University of Nevada–Las Vegas granted the second author a President's Fellowship during the last year of her graduate training, and this assistance greatly facilitated our work. Finally, we would like to thank our husbands, Tim and Dominic, for their emotional support and intellectual contributions during data collection and manuscript preparation. Thank you all. We are deeply appreciative.

Obesity Surgery

Introduction

If I only had the heart, the brain, the nerve . . .
—THE WIZARD OF OZ

Six years ago, we attended a prospective-patient seminar on gastric bypass surgery. Our training in health psychology had made us a little skeptical of surgical interventions for behavioral problems, but we wanted to learn more about the procedure and the people who were considering it. Sure, we were aware that, for some folks, obesity was partly genetic. We knew that only a minority of dieters maintained their weight loss. Clearly, the whole enterprise was difficult, yet eating and lifestyles remained behaviors amenable to change. We were believers in the power of psychological interventions, of will-power buttressed by emotional support and solid behavioral techniques.

Sitting among the audience of severely obese individuals and a smattering of significant others, we found ourselves humbled by the challenges these individuals had faced in the past and were about to confront in their near future. As we walked back to the parking lot and drove to our offices at the University of Nevada—Las Vegas, our discussion veered far from the concerns we had brought to the seminar. We didn't discuss whether this surgery was really necessary or whether these folks would be better served by a good lifestyle-modification program. We wondered what their lives were like and the ways in which these lives would be changed by weight loss. Six years ago we went looking for a story about losing weight and found a story about finding self—a story about what happens when you get rid of the one thing you are convinced is standing between you and your dreams.

Obese or not, most of us have at some point wished we could change something about ourselves. We fantasize about how much better our lives would be if we could just make some significant adjustments to our looks, our finances, our careers. Entire industries are built on our chronic dissatisfaction with ourselves and our lives. Reality television also nurtures our self-dissatisfaction and our fantasies about the consequences of radical "self-improvement." Transformations are elusive, though. Most of us are left tinkering with minor alterations and daydreaming about the happiness that might have been ours had we been able to fulfill a wish. But what happens when this wish comes true? Would our lives really be easier or better if we became transformed—reborn?

The people we met at that obesity-surgery seminar were banking on it. They were willing to risk their lives (at the time, the surgery had a higher death rate)[1] to finally experience some positive life changes they had long fantasized about. The extent to which the reality of living on the "greener" side of the fence measured up to these fantasies was the question that interested us. The surgery would make them lose weight, but would the weight loss result in the fulfillment of those preoperative wishes?

In one way, the odds looked pretty good to us. Losing weight would surely improve many aspects of these individuals' lives—they would be healthier, have more mobility, feel more attractive, and so on. The list seemed endless. We live in a society that is openly prejudicial and cruel to people who are clinically obese. Losing a significant amount of weight seemed likely to result in dramatically positive changes both in self-perception and in the perceptions of others. However, we also had a sense it might get a little complicated. As psychologists, we started our research knowing too much about psychological processes to ever expect the surgery to be a fix-all. There are no fix-alls.

So six years ago when obesity surgery was pretty rare, we set out to ask a simple question that no one had asked before. How did your life change when you lost anywhere from 85 to 350 pounds? Was it what you thought it would be? Obesity surgery represents one of those rare opportunities in life in which we get to shed the part of ourselves that we dislike and for which the world discriminates against us. How does all that play out? The question is more relevant now than ever in regards to weight loss, simply because so many more people are opting for the surgery.

Over the years during which we conducted our research, we saw the popularity of obesity surgery skyrocket, partly as a function of the following:

1   media attention

2   the normalizing impact of celebrity disclosures

3   technological advances in obesity surgery

4   a growing concern about the rise in obesity in the United States (currently one third of American adults are obese, and 5 percent are severely obese)[2]

At the time of our first interviews, there were no Carnie Wilson, Al Roker, Randy Jackson, or Sharon Osbourne celebrity disclosures. It was by no means the topic of television newsmagazines and print articles. The situation was quite the opposite. There seemed to be a cloak of secrecy surrounding the procedure. The general perception was that it was a desperate move reserved for individuals practically on their deathbed because of obesity. All of that has changed dramatically.

It is estimated that in 2005, 170,000 weight loss surgeries were performed in the United States—nearly five times as many as in 2000.[3] These numbers are expected to continue to rise. Between 1998 and 2002, the number of bariatric (the word *bariatric* refers to the branch of medicine dealing with the causes, prevention, and treatment of obesity) surgeons in the American Society for Bariatric Surgery rose from 258 to 641.[4] Research on obesity surgery has also grown exponentially, as have patient-support services. Accompanying the growth in popularity have been remarkable advances in surgical technology, especially in regard to laparoscopic procedures. In contrast to traditional "open" surgery, which involves a large incision through the midsection, these procedures involve tiny incisions sufficient to allow the entry of the surgical instruments and a camera.[5] Such procedures significantly reduce complications and recovery periods. The introduction of the Lap-Band procedure has also revolutionized obesity surgery by providing the option of constricting the stomach by way of a band, rather than surgical reduction.[6] The band is designed to be adjustable to varying levels of constriction, and, if necessary, it can be removed altogether.

Despite the general boom in obesity surgery over the past six years, a sprinkling of more sobering stories is surfacing. Recently, patients have started speaking out about the emotional and psychological complexities of life after surgery and dramatic weight loss:

- Al Roker cried on national television discussing the emotional process that accompanies the surgery and weight loss,

- The May 16, 2005, issue of *New York* magazine featured an article on how stomach surgery "gets you thin but not necessarily happy"

- The *Pittsburgh Post Gazette* of June 29, 2005, printed an article on how gastric bypass surgery patients often find "it's not a cure for depression"

Comedian Jessica Fisher has a stand-up comedy act available on DVD that delves into the unanticipated ways in which dramatic weight loss changed her life.

Weight loss surgery is clearly very effective at helping people lose enormous amounts of weight, but it does not fix all the problems in their lives. Through our interviews we learned that it might even create some. That is not an argument against the surgery, but rather a precaution. It may not be the panacea or all-encompassing solution that many people expect it to be. There is also an alarming trend to regain weight approximately two years after the procedure. What leads to this regain? We think the answer might be in the extent to which individuals are able to successfully navigate the psychological, emotional, and relational challenges that the surgery and weight loss pose.

We were fortunate to make the acquaintance of an exceptionally psychologically minded bariatric surgeon practicing in Las Vegas, Dr. Barry Fisher. Dr. Fisher was as concerned with the psychological and social lives of his patients as with the physiological outcome of his surgical handiwork. His thinking was that if the quality of life of his patients did not significantly improve after surgery, they would eventually regain the weight. He was not interested in simply helping people lose weight in the short run—he sincerely wanted to improve the lives of his patients holistically.

Obesity-surgery patients remain on a very restrictive diet after the procedure, and they need to have sufficient motivation to adhere to the difficult diet.[7] This seems a little ironic, since most of them had not dieted successfully prior to the surgery. Why would they be successful now? Together with Dr. Fisher, we suspected the answer might be in the improved quality of their lives. The surgery gave the weight loss a big kick-start. As the weight started to drop, patients would experience significant improvements in their lives. These improvements would then provide the motivational fuel that made them stick to their diet.

We are grateful that Dr. Fisher wished to collaborate with psychologists who were as interested as he was in the ways in which his patients coped with the consequences of weight loss. Because of his profound interest in the psychological and social outcome of this surgery, we were given access to the world of his patients. They, in turn, gave generously of their time and privacy to allow us to piece together what happened before and after they left the operating room and returned to surprisingly altered lives.

We conducted in-depth individual and group interviews with twenty-four women and nine men. The fact that the majority of patients we accessed were women is no accident—it reflects the gender ratio of individuals who seek to have obesity surgery. Despite the fact that just as many women as men in the United States are severely obese, 80 percent of weight loss–surgery patients are women.[8] The reasons for this discrepancy have not yet been determined in any scientific way. It seems likely that the gender difference is attributable to one of several potential reasons: Women tend to seek help for personal and health problems more frequently than men;[9] severe obesity can interfere substantially with one's ability to parent children, and women tend to be the primary caregivers; or men suffer fewer detriments to self-image and less societal discrimination than women do as a function of being grossly overweight.[10] Perhaps it is a combination of all of these factors that results in the overrepresentation of women in obesity surgery.

Our youngest interviewee was thirty years old, and our oldest was fifty-

three, with the average age of the group at forty-one years. All were heterosexual. Thirty were European American (Caucasian), and two were Hispanic
American. There was a mix of married, divorced, and single individuals,
and just over half of them had children. We interviewed people with a variety of occupations, including stay-at-home moms, entrepreneurs, teachers,
clerical workers, attorneys, architects, students, nurses, security guards, real
estate professionals, hairdressers, and a couple of individuals who were un-
employed at the time of the interview. Many walks of life and income levels
were represented in our group.

All of our interviewees underwent Roux-n-Y gastric bypass surgery. There
was a fair amount of variation in terms of preoperative weight, weight lost at
time of interview, and time passed since the surgery. The preoperative weight
of the individuals we interviewed ranged from 225 to 525 pounds, with the
average being 372 pounds.

- 17 percent of the group had a preoperative weight of under 300 pounds
- 46 percent weighed between 300 and 400 pounds
- 37 percent had weighed more than 400 pounds at the time of surgery
- three individuals weighed more than 500 pounds preoperatively

Weight lost at the time of interview ranged from 85 pounds to 350 pounds,
with the average weight lost at the time of interview being 177 pounds. Time
since surgery ranged from six months to ten years, but the majority of the
folks we interviewed (60 percent) were less than three years out of surgery.
Two of our interviewees had had the surgery ten years previous. We thus
had the perspective of lightweights and heavyweights, rookies and veterans.
However, it is important to note that our sample of people was considerably
heavier than the average person seeking or considering obesity surgery today. Although the lightweights in our study tended to experience less dramatic life changes with the weight loss, the changes tended to occur in the
same domains with similar, though perhaps less intense, effects.

We asked all of these folks the same basic open-ended question: In what
ways has your life changed consequent to the weight loss after obesity sur-

gery? Their answers were rich and varied. Most started by telling us what their lives were like before the surgery and what drove them to opt for the procedure. We taped all the interviews and transcribed them. We then read over each one carefully, and, using a methodology called "grounded theory," we coded the interviews for the emergence of certain themes—some were common to many interviewees, and some were unique to an individual.[11] We then put all of these data together to construct an overall picture of what generally happened to folks before and, in more detail, after the surgery. Toward the end of the book we present a theory of how we think the consequences of the surgery may be related to long-term outcomes. In the last chapter, we propose a series of steps to help those who opt for obesity surgery prepare for and cope with the many changes they will face.

Through this methodology, we hope to communicate the complexity and richness of these individuals' experiences as faithfully as possible. No two individuals reported an identical experience. However, their stories gave us a definite sense that there was a commonality of experience that speaks to universal concerns about the construction of self and how our sense of who we are is shaped by our relationships, both superficial and intimate.

In order to protect the confidentiality of the individuals we interviewed, we changed their names and any other potentially identifying details in their quotes. We also occasionally edited the quotes to correct normal grammatical errors made in speech or to shorten the length of a particular story. Other than in the case of these minimal changes, every quote is taken verbatim from the transcripts of the interviews we conducted.

An obvious omission in the chapters that follow is the struggle to maintain the strict dietary regimen necessitated by the surgery. Many people uninformed in the realities of obesity surgery think that this reconfigured tiny stomach or newly constricted passage eliminates cravings for the types and portions of food that are likely to result in weight gain. This is not true. As Carnie Wilson's book title, *I Am Still Hungry!* so aptly states, obesity surgery is a tool that greatly facilitates weight loss and reduced consumption, but it does not eliminate cravings. Providing further evidence of this, Wilson was a guest on a television show in which celebrities who want to lose weight compete with each other to do so. And, in her case, this was years after having had weight loss surgery!

As mentioned previously, a significant number of people start regaining the weight approximately two years after the surgery. This regain has typically been attributed to a failure to maintain the postoperative dietary regimen. Although the capacity of the stomach is significantly reduced, it can accommodate grazing (snacking continuously throughout the day) and poor food choices. This book has purposefully avoided the topic of postsurgical diets. Central though the postsurgical dietary struggle is, we were specifically interested in the life changes that may make the required, lifelong dieting worth it or not. There are other resources that offer dietary advice, and we provide a list of them at the end of this text.

A brief summary of the lessons the men and women in this book taught us has already been published in the academic press[12] and has been presented at national and international conferences.[13] However, none of these abbreviated forms of communication gave us the opportunity to make the interviewees' voices widely heard and with all the richness and detail we had listened to. In the next few chapters, we pass the microphone back over to them.

Part 1

Getting There from Here

CHAPTER 1 | **Taking the Leap**

Deciding on Surgery

I don't want to die—I'm worth living.
—DAPHNE

If you stood on a street corner at rush hour in any American city today and asked every passerby whether they would like to lose some weight, most would say yes. If you then asked them why, people would smile and say either to look better or to be healthier. Losing weight would be nice, and it makes an annual appearance on their lists of New Year's resolutions. For a smaller group of severely obese people, the situation is considerably more drastic. They would report that weight stands squarely between them and their dreams. Some might even tell you that their lives are hanging in the balance. That is precisely the case for the ten to fifteen million Americans who are severely obese. When you weigh 100 or more pounds than you should, there are as many reasons to want to lose weight as there are excess pounds— and they are all compelling, if not urgent. Clinically severe obesity can destroy your body, threaten the integrity of your self-concept, play havoc with careers and relationships, and make you an outsider in a society openly dismissive of people who look like you.

Severe obesity has been linked with five of the ten leading causes of death in the United States, including heart disease, some types of cancer, stroke, diabetes, and atherosclerosis.[1] Hypertension and high cholesterol are par for the course. Other potentially incapacitating conditions include chronic fatigue, severe sleep apnea and sleep deprivation, respiratory problems, chronic

pain, edema (swelling), erosive skin rashes, incontinence, and immune deficiencies resulting in frequent bouts of the flu, colds, and infections. Generally,
the more severe the obesity, the more serious the medical complications and
the higher the mortality risk. The term *morbid obesity* is meant to link extreme obesity to the many health risks it poses, as the word *morbid* simply
means diseased.

Individuals who are extremely obese are also seriously affected emotionally and psychologically. Depression and anxiety are common. Low self-
esteem and self-confidence, as well as difficulty being assertive, are widely
reported. The usually lifelong struggle to lose weight and maintain the loss
often results in eating-disordered behavior, primarily bingeing and grazing
(snacking continuously). Relationships also pose a significant challenge for
many severely obese individuals. There seems to be an increased tendency
to stay in relationships that are less than satisfactory or even abusive. The
reason for this may lie in the belief that they are lucky to have been able to
attract anyone at all. Some morbidly obese people give up on relationships
altogether, not believing a healthy one possible, given their appearance and
doubts about self and others. They may be suspicious of anyone who wants
to be with them a la Groucho Marx, who didn't want to be a member of
any club that would admit him as a member. This is not to say that severely
obese individuals cannot find fulfilling relationships. They can and they do,
but they may be facing an even more daunting challenge than the rest of the
population. Finally, as a function of their physical limitations, obese individuals often lead highly inactive and isolated lives. Making it from one room
of the house to another without resting may be questionable, and going out
socially is often completely out of the question.

Adding insult to injury is a society so unforgiving of obesity that there
is often barely an attempt to disguise the discrimination and harassment.
Because weight gain is widely believed to be controllable, obesity is often
considered a sign of character weakness.[2] This popular point of view seems
to grant the general public permission to be explicitly unkind to obese individuals. The open and unabashed stigmatization of obesity has been described as the "last safe prejudice" in American society.[3] Even children have

described silhouettes of an obese child as lazy, stupid, and deceptive and rated them as least likable in a series of silhouettes of all types of children, including those with other serious disabilities.[4] So either we are socializing children to reject overweight individuals on essentially moral grounds, or maybe someone would venture the argument that we are genetically pre-disposed to ostracize those among us who are different.[5] It's hard to know. Either way, evidence for what looks like obesity discrimination has been found in college entrance rates, hiring practices, socioeconomic upward mo-bility, and, shockingly, even in the attitudes of health-care providers.[6]

So morbid obesity packs a triple punch. You may be in seriously bad shape physically, the richness of your life may be shrinking before your very eyes, and you live in a society that every day finds old and novel ways to tell you that you are among the most undesirable of its citizens. How's that for mo-tivation to change your life by whatever means possible? Pretty compelling, one would think, yet virtually all of the people we interviewed had been se-verely obese for many, many years before deciding on the surgery. They had first tried all types of interventions, from every imaginable diet to prescrip-tion diet pills to street-bought amphetamines. Their battle with weight had been lifelong and unsuccessful, as it is for the vast majority of severely obese individuals.

Nationally, only 5 percent of individuals struggling with extreme obesity who try nonsurgical methods keep the weight off for a significant amount of time.[7] An even smaller number keep it off for good. And those discouraging weight loss outcomes are not just a characteristic of obese dieters. Weight loss techniques cycle in and out of fashion, temporarily generating gargan-tuan profits for the latest strategy, be that a low-carbohydrate, low-fat, or just liquid diet. The fact that the diet market is so huge is an indication of both our preoccupation with weight loss and the ultimate failure of most of our attempts. When one strategy fails to work, you invest in another. One large-scale survey found that, in the United States, one out of every three men and one out of every two women were trying to lose weight. The minority of peo-ple who succeed in achieving weight loss will regain nearly two-thirds of it within one year, and all of it will be regained five years after the initial weight loss.[8] So losing weight and keeping it off for the long haul are extremely difficult for everyone.

For the severely obese, weight loss surgery thus becomes the only alternative that holds any hope. There are a number of different types of weight loss surgeries, but they all basically entail surgically altering the gastrointestinal system so that less food can be consumed or absorbed or both. Although these surgeries are far more popular and less invasive than they were twenty years ago, they are still major surgical procedures that dramatically alter the way the body works. An unprecedented number of people are opting for these surgeries today, but these procedures are still viewed by most overweight people as a last resort, when all other methods of weight loss have failed them. The recent exponential rise in weight loss surgeries has prompted some experts to worry that individuals who could have gained control of their weight by other noninvasive methods are jumping into the operating room all too eagerly. This type of premature eagerness did not seem to characterize the people we interviewed. Most of them felt truly desperate about their situation and simply could not conceive of any other recourse, despite significant fears about the procedure. They saw no other alternative. Virtually all the people we interviewed decided to have the surgery at what they described as a point of despair.

> DAPHNE: *I remember I had stepped on the scale, and I saw how heavy I was [350 pounds]. I was taking a shower with my kids who were toddlers at the time. Now this is a small square shower, and I pretty much took up the whole space. I remember crying hard and looking up and crunching my fists and saying, "Why? God, why are you letting me die? I'm a good person. I do everything I can for anybody I can. Why are you just taking me away from who I want to be and what I want to be? Why won't you help me?" And I just continued to cry, and I was pretty much yelling at God. And I remember saying, "I've asked you over and over to help me, and you won't help me. If you are God, if you are real, I need to know that, and I need you to help me."*

This feeling of powerlessness over the weight was typical. Contrary to popular views of obese individuals as not caring about their weight, our interviewees had waged strong campaigns against their weight at different times of their lives. They had vacillated between periods of extreme dieting to periods of giving up entirely and sinking into the multidimensional havoc that the weight wreaked. The weight seemed to have a life of its own over which they exerted little control. The extent to which this feeling of power-lessness was an accurate reflection of their actual power to change their bodies and their lives is hard to know. It is clear, though, that the surgery was a last resort primarily because of how long they each took to actually decide to go ahead with it. Most had resisted this decision for a very long time. We did not see much evidence of cavalier jumps into this procedure, although some obesity-surgery patients do enter into that decision relatively uninformed.[9]

Resisting the Last Resort

Why didn't they do it before? Why did they wait so long and suffer so much before undergoing the only intervention that seemed to stand a chance of succeeding? It is a question we can all ask ourselves about any aspect of our lives we have let deteriorate to near irreparability before taking action—from an abusive relationship to a dead-end job to a life-robbing substance dependence. It is a question central to our understanding of when and how human beings change their circumstances. Health professionals and behavioral scientists have yet to answer it in any satisfactory way. This question came to haunt many of the people who actually succeeded in making the change, as they pined postoperatively for lost time and opportunities.

> BRANDON: *What I find amazing and have no answer for is why I and other people let themselves get to this sorry point. I wish I had done it earlier because there were a lot of wasted years as a result of being heavy and not being able to do things.*

Most people who engage in self-destructive behavior know they are harming themselves. That is why public health campaigns focusing on the damage people are inflicting on themselves are simply not very effective.[10] Try telling a smoker that his or her behavior could lead to lung cancer or emphysema. Virtually no smoker of sound mind today is unaware that it is harmful to them. So knowing something is bad for us may be necessary in order to stop doing it, but that knowledge alone is nowhere near enough. Why is that? The answer is quite simple. It is easier to continue doing what we are doing than to try to stop. But at what cost, you ask? That is a question every individual has to answer for themselves. For some people the cost can be death itself, as in the case of heroin addicts who know that every hit carries the risk of a fatal overdose. For others, such as smokers, it is the looming threat of life-threatening illnesses in the future. For people who are severely obese, it is anything from a sudden stroke to heart disease to diabetes, not to mention the mounting limitations on everyday activities and relationships.

Our interviewees had reached a turning point at which they had decided the cost of being obese had become prohibitive. This turning point was rarely characterized by a single event. Most had suffered the consequences of being extremely obese for many years. Although these consequences were getting graver with age, there did not seem to be any cataclysmic event or realization that drove them to seek help. Rather, it seemed to be more of an accumulation of frustration with the mounting limitations on their lives. They all seemed to hit rock bottom at some point, and a voice inside suddenly said, "That's enough." Many were able to describe their reasons for holding out and not taking the steps needed to lose the weight. Their accounts provide important information about the mystery surrounding inaction in the face of such difficult circumstances.

Fear of Surgery and Mistrust of Doctors

The most common reason given to us for delaying the decision to have surgery was fear of the procedure. And who is not fearful of surgery, even the simplest outpatient procedure? Grown men without a pound of excess fat have been known to shudder at the prospect of it. Surgery always carries some risk, and, as one of our interviewees, Lawrence, emphasized, "This is no run-of-the-mill appendectomy." Gastric bypass surgery (laparoscopic or not) is a lengthy and delicate surgical procedure that can result in serious postoperative complications and even death. Furthermore, these procedures are doubly complicated by the fact that they are performed on people who are often in relatively poor health at the time. When you are out of breath just getting out of bed to go to the bathroom, it is easy to imagine why you might be terrified of going under the knife. Brandon expressed that at 525 pounds he was "fully prepared not to survive the surgery."

This fear of major surgery, natural to most people regardless of their weight or health status, is compounded in the severely obese person by a common and profound distrust of the medical profession. A number of our interviewees complained of their treatment over the years at the hands of doctors.

> URSULA: *I was dismissed in emergency rooms because I was fat. What I was saying was discounted. No matter what was wrong with me, all they would ever say is, "You need to lose the weight, and you'll be fine."*

Much like the rest of the world, there are doctors who look at obese people and see only the weight. Our interviewees believed that the weight literally blinded health care professionals to any other health problem they might be experiencing. It appears that health care professionals are not immune to prejudice against the severely obese, as some research studies have shown. The ultimate effect is that some of our interviewees despaired of ever being listened to by doctors who could not get past the excess pounds.

> RONALD: *Every doctor I've gone to, every ER, regardless of my problem, they don't get past the weight. I fell down, hurt my back. I fell off the top of a mixer truck onto a concrete block. And the only test this doctor wanted to do was an EKG [electrocardiogram]. I found out in a lot of instances they just want to do EKGs. They automatically assume that it is a weight problem, not anything else. Their only focus is on your weight.*

It may seem natural for health professionals to focus on the weight of the clinically severely obese patient. After all, health professionals are acutely aware of the health consequences and risks involved. Research has also shown that when doctors tell patients they are concerned about some aspect of their health behavior, patients are more likely to attempt behavior change.[11]

But one can also understand the frustration of the obese patient who can't get flu medication without hearing the familiar lecture. These patients were hearing nothing new when the doctor cataloged all the reasons the weight was dangerous. They knew that already. Lack of information was not their problem. The admonishing lectures they had repeatedly gotten from doctors, no matter the nature of their presenting complaint, had not resulted in weight loss. It had resulted in a dangerous avoidance of health professionals, who had come to be perceived by many of our interviewees as punishing rather than helpful.

> MAGGIE: *I didn't trust doctors. The doctors I went to before said, "It's your fault. You could lose this weight if you wanted to." One actually said, "You're just stupid." When I was pregnant with my son and going into labor, my doctor (whom I was moderately comfortable with) had broken his arm, so another gentleman stepped in. This substitute doctor had never seen me. He came in, and I was extremely heavy [more than 400 pounds], extremely pregnant, and he took one look at me and said, "Oh, God, I've got this one?!" And I'm lying there in pain on the table, and he says, "Prep her for a c-section—she's never going to have that child the normal way." I became very visibly upset, and the nurse calmed me down and said, "Don't worry about it. He's going to be gone for a while—we'll get you through this." The nurses were the greatest—they saved me. I had that child before the doctor came back, and I had him the natural way. And I heard him say when he returned, "Well, I didn't think she could do it."*

The frustration with physicians thus seemed to emanate from what felt like a discriminatory attitude in which all physical problems were automatically attributed to weight. It felt like a dismissal, if not an outright put-down. The insult of this perfunctory and offensive treatment was probably compounded by the fact that the doctors typically did not provide any suggestions that resulted in effective weight loss. If doctors were so sure weight was the source of all medical problems, how come they couldn't suggest any potential solutions? Why didn't they know that dieting alone just did not work? Why did they, who were supposed to be educated, also act as if obesity was simply a reflection of weakness of character and lack of will? It felt like a medical "throwing up of the hands" and a dumping of the problem on the laps of these individuals. As we mentioned previously, information alone is not sufficient to make people change their behavior. People need skills. They need help with the "how-to."

So these types of experiences made our interviewees turn to doctors only in cases of extreme necessity. The decision to have weight loss surgery would involve entering into a long-term relationship with a profession by which they had felt mistreated and betrayed. Even if the reason for seeing a doctor this time was precisely about weight and weight alone, many of our interviewees said it took them a long time to trust that any doctor, even an obesity surgeon, would actually really care what happened to them. Ironically, doctors felt dangerous even to some of our very ill interviewees.

Hopelessness and Shame

Self-defeatism was another reason that had kept some of our interviewees from opting for the surgery for as long as they did. They thought their situation was hopeless. They had trouble believing that even this surgery could get rid of the weight they had struggled with, for as long as they could remember. At 350 pounds, Daphne felt she was "a lost cause." After so many years of failing to lose or even maintain their already high weight, the interviewees' temptation to simply give up on any intervention seemed natural. Why get hopeful and set yourself up for yet another disappointment? As Brandon put it, "I didn't think the operation was going to work—nothing else had."

There was also a significant amount of shame in the thought of choosing surgery. Although weight loss surgery and the lifelong dietary regimen mandated are anything but easy, many of our interviewees reported being criticized for "taking the easy way out." Frances remembers her cousin (also overweight) saying to her, "Look at what you are thinking of doing, and I am still fighting the real fight. You are taking the easy way out, and look at what you are resorting to." And although our interviewees knew the surgery, the postoperative recovery, and the lifelong dieting ahead would be very challenging, they reported that they had felt somewhat ashamed to have the surgery. They admitted that, at moments, they had wished they could shout to the world that they were losing the weight "all on their own." So part of the shame in deciding on the surgery emanated from an internalized sense of failure.

But there was also another source of shame. Frances felt that the surgery itself was a clear sign of desperation and that showing the world that desperation was itself embarrassing.

FRANCES: *That somebody does this is proof of how desperate they are, and maybe I just didn't want anybody to ever see that. The knowledge of that desperation is something so private, so personal . . .*

It is important for all of us to save face with the people around us and even with ourselves. Admitting we have a problem can feel humiliating, so we often tell people and ourselves that we are okay with our supposed problem, that it doesn't really bother us, that it does not define us or even really affect us. If we are obese and think it is inconceivable to lose weight, we might as well act as if it does not matter to us. At the very least, we won't feel that we are disclosing our personal pain to others. Deciding to have the surgery is a kind of "coming out"—it is a way of telling the world that, yes, it does bother us, we feel powerless over the problem, and it's gotten bad enough for us to do something relatively dramatic to change it. This "coming out" is tough because it requires us to tolerate the vulnerability of admitting to the world that we want to be something other than what we are. It is, thus, hardly surprising that people engage in a certain amount of denial.

Denial and Resignation

Often a barrier to change, denial is sometimes difficult to separate from a healthy acceptance of things outside of our control. To some extent, we are all in denial about something. We certainly are not all confronting and addressing all of the problems in our lives. Are we in denial about these problems, or are we just trying to live as best we can, given a set of circumstances and limitations? It's hard to say. Denial is always assessed either by someone outside the situation (our family, our friends, or our doctor) or by us only *after* we have made some change. Denial is for the most part a hindsight judgment.

A handful of our interviewees actually said that prior to the surgery they had not considered themselves to be *that* heavy. Others claimed to have made realistic assessments of their weight—they knew they were very heavy—but they had resigned themselves to living with the obesity. "I always thought, this will do—my little life," laughed Karina, as she recalled her attitude presurgery at 445 pounds. My little life! Karina's three-word description of her presurgical world succinctly communicates resignation, if not full-on denial. She was admitting that her life was "little," but she had convinced herself that "little" was good enough. She had even managed to make it sound cute and accommodating. This type of convincing ourselves that a less-than-full life would be sufficient was very common in the mind-set of our interviewees prior to reaching their turning point.

> ORIANNA: *I had a man who loved me and a home and puppies, and I had myself believing it was okay, that . . . this was what life was all about, this is what it was going to be for me and it was okay, that I could live the rest of my life like this. And when my family would say, "We worry you're not going to live till you're fifty," I'd say, "Well, if I die, that's okay."*

At 500 pounds, Orianna had even made peace with the thought that she might die young. She had accommodated to the point of being "okay" with dying before the age of fifty! Others even tried to put a positive individualistic spin on their obesity, as if it were a unique characteristic that distinguished them from others.

> PENELOPE: *I had accepted at a certain point that I was going to be a large person [240 pounds preop]. I had gone through a certain point in my development at which I thought, "Well, I guess Penelope is one of those people that is going to walk around a little bigger than the rest of the world." And I could accept being different. And that was cool, 'cause I'm a different kind of person on the inside. It's the way I'm wired.*

These folks had convinced themselves, for better or for worse, that who they were and what they had were all they could hope for. They told themselves they could be satisfied with the status quo. Research on behavior change shows that there are five different stages people go through before deciding to take the difficult step of changing their behavior.[12] The first of these stages is the precontemplation stage, in which we have no intention of changing the behavior in question. At this stage, most of us don't even admit we have a problem. We may make some attempts to fix it, out of pressure from family members or friends, but most of these attempts fail because we are not truly motivated to change yet. The contemplation stage is when we become aware that we have a problem, start thinking of making changes, but have not yet committed to it. This is the familiar "Gee, I really should do something about my weight" or "I really should stop smoking" stage. The contemplation stage can last years, during which we seem to be weighing the pros and cons of the behavior yet continue to focus more on the pros than the cons. The preparation stage is when we start actually making plans to change. We might make a deadline for actually seeking help or stopping the behavior. We may be waiting for a stressful event to pass before engaging in the change, but we seem to have decided that we are going to do it. Usually, in the preparation stage we already start modifying our behavior, as in eating a little less or smoking fewer cigarettes. In the fourth stage, action, we start engaging in behavior change. Finally, there is the maintenance stage in which we work to prevent relapse. People in denial are generally considered to be in the precontemplation stage or contemplation stage, and some of our interviewees said they remained in this stage for a long time. They were plainly trying to accept their weight as part of who they were or choosing to focus on the positive aspects of the status quo.

One fascinating manifestation of this acceptance was an outright lack of a physical image of self. Some folks reported that when they were heavy, they had no picture in their mind of what they looked like. Once they lost the weight, they still did not have a mental picture of themselves as physical beings. Their self-image was centered on their inner selves and not on their shells—their bodies.

ABBY: *I've never had a physical image of myself in my mind. I was just Abby, and when I saw my picture, my before-the-surgery picture [367 pounds], I didn't know I looked like that. And when I see myself now [117 pounds], I still do not have an image of how I look. I just see Abby. I just see who I am in my mind.*

Thus, one way of coping seemed to be to self-identify in ways other than via appearance, a domain that was clearly not going to be esteem enhancing for our group. It seems like a good defense to place our self-esteem in an area that is likely to be appreciated rather than in an area we know we do not excel in. But over and above coping, don't most of us claim to value what people carry inside rather than how they look? Is that not what we teach our children? Haven't we seen movies such as the *Elephant Man* and *Mask* and felt elevated by the fact that under the unattractive shell lived a gem to be uncovered by people with a little bit of depth? Most people would agree that what really matters in a person are qualities such as kindness or integrity or intelligence, yet severely obese individuals will tell you that has not been their experience. Only a few people got past their looks to find out who they really were. Consequently, some of our interviewees created a self-concept that did not include their physical appearance. Whether this was a defense to fend off the painful fact of their obesity or not, this lack of a physical self-concept persisted after the surgery, even when it was no longer as useful as it once had been.

So, in one sense, resigning ourselves to circumstances that appear hard to change may not be a bad coping strategy—insofar as our judgment of what can be changed and what can't remains accurate. And therein lies the rub!

RONALD: *You know it just became part of life. You don't realize what you are doing to yourself. You really don't. You feel like you're okay. Just because somebody has a problem with your weight [447 pounds], makes fun of you or whatever, it's been such a pattern through your life that you just think that's the way it is.*

On the other hand, this type of learned helplessness can result in depression, suicidality, and illness.[13] People who feel they have lost all control over adverse things happening to them do not tend to do well psychologically or physically. It is a risky coping strategy to give up trying to improve our lives when we aren't happy. The other problem with the resignation and acceptance strategy is that most of our interviewees did not stop gaining weight at the time of their acceptance. They continued putting on the pounds and accumulating the health complications. Giving up did not mean stabilizing at a certain high weight. The status quo was a shifting target that demanded an increasing accommodation to negative circumstances. To what lengths could they maintain their "This is not really bothering me" stance? Just when they thought they had become accustomed to not being able to do something, another "something" became impossible. Just as they had finally accommodated one loss, another loss came knocking. Life was asking them to continue accepting a constantly expanding list of negative outcomes. The degenerative aspect of their situation begged a question of most of our interviewees, "Where is my limit?"

Saying Good-bye to Food

The decision to have weight loss surgery was very different from simply going on another diet that we could drop on Friday and start again on Monday. Gastric bypass surgery is permanent and requires saying good-bye to eating what we want, when we want it, in whatever quantity we desire. It means committing to a lifetime of restrained eating—and many of our interviewees just weren't sure if they were up to the challenge. Most of them were veteran dieters. If there was a diet out there, they had tried it. Most of them had lost a lot of weight on various diets several times throughout their lives. The kicker was that these diets were impossible to maintain for long, and when they stopped dieting, the weight came back—and then some. Our interviewees were not convinced they could succeed at the one thing they had failed at all of their lives: dieting. The very thought of being on yet another diet made most of them cringe. It was a cross they had long ago decided they could no longer bear.

PENELOPE: *I had dropped my diet consciousness. I didn't want to "be" a diet anymore. I would have to "be" a diet again.*

Penelope's intentional reference to herself as a "diet" rather than as "someone on a diet" powerfully conveys the near obsessive thinking and behavior necessary to stay committed to losing weight. Dieting can easily become an all-consuming endeavor. When you are not eating, you are thinking about food and how you can't have any. When you *are* eating, you have to think carefully about what and how much. The gimmick to most diets—whether of the low-fat, low-carbohydrate, liquid, grapefruit, or cabbage-soup variety—is that they all involve a dramatic reduction in overall caloric intake. There is no question that maintaining a low caloric intake will make you lose weight, but at what cost?

The effects of starvation diets have been well documented. Most notorious perhaps is the work by Ancel Keys and colleagues at the University of Minnesota, conducted more than fifty years ago.[14] Keys, considered a public health icon for his many contributions to the scientific community, set out to study the effects of starvation. He and his researchers watched closely as healthy men (conscientious objectors) were put on a semistarvation diet for three months. Their calories were cut in half. The men experienced significant deterioration in their psychological and social well-being. It is important to note here that this "semistarvation" experiment involved consuming many more calories per day than the kind of conservative diets prescribed to obese people today.[15] Weighing in daily, counting calories, and reading product labels can become a tyranny that people experience as oppressive. If you add to that the psychological effects of starvation, individuals simply find themselves thinking about little else besides food. You *become* a diet, as Penelope says.

Other people in our study said their reluctance to have surgery grew out of a fear of not being able to beat what they considered their *addiction* to food. There are strong differences in opinion among experts about whether overeating constitutes a true addiction, but there is also little question that overeating and substance dependence share some similar characteristics.[16] Many of our interviewees were convinced that they were addicted to food the way other people are addicted to drugs or alcohol. To further complicate matters, breaking an "addiction" to food is very different from breaking an addiction to substances, because you cannot make a clean break with food the way you can with alcohol or drugs.

> MAGGIE: *It's an addiction. I mean people smoke; they can't stop. People drink; they can't stop. You've got those people who don't drink or smoke who tell you, "You could quit if you wanted to." Drugs are very simple to get on. I mean, they make you feel good, just like food made me feel. It was a comfort. It didn't criticize me; it just fed me. It made my stomach feel warm; it made me feel warm. But the problem here is that you can quit cigarettes, but you can't quit food.*

Maggie raises an important point here, as abstinence is the mainstay of most addiction programs. The message in addiction rehabilitation is, with few exceptions, "You can never touch the stuff again, because you have shown you have no control once you start." Well, that is just not possible with food. So for those of our interviewees who believed they were addicted to food, moderate eating posed the same challenge that moderate substance use would to a substance addict—a very difficult or, according to some, close-to-impossible challenge.

The Turning Points

For the people we interviewed, each of the aforementioned reasons for not having the surgery was at some point overpowered by an accumulation of life insults. One last painful consequence of their obesity had changed their minds, their hearts, their wills. Their own proverbial line in the sand appeared before them. They had all decided they would not cross that line. They all knew that whatever rationalizations they had been telling themselves to resist having surgery were no longer convincing. They knew something had to be done, that they could not continue as they had for so long. Frances strongly believes that desperation is actually a prerequisite to a successful outcome: "You know, when a patient gets to the point where they are signing the consent for the surgery, if they are not desperate, they do not belong in this situation."

According to Frances and a number of the other interviewees, it is the desperation that is motivating. The concept of desperation is often invoked as a motivating force that leads to bad decisions. We talk about people choosing a bad romantic partner or making risky financial investments out of desperation, as if desperation invariably leads to bad judgment. We say no to a number of offers in our lives by proudly stating, "Thanks, but I am not that desperate!" But desperation also has its upside. It can mean that we have reached a point at which it becomes crystal clear what we will and will not accept in our lives. A number of clichés refer to that point: do or die, back up against a wall, hitting rock bottom. You are either going to stay down there, or you are going to pick yourself up and turn things around. Desperation can also lead to creative solutions that did not seem viable until the desperation set in. Ergo, another cliché: Necessity is the mother of invention. So desperation is both something we fear and are ashamed of as well as a shining opportunity for change, dismal though it may feel at the time. Many of our interviewees believed that after the surgery, it was the memory of that terrible desperation that fueled their drive to cope with the challenging struggles ahead. They simply never wanted to feel that way again.

> JESSICA: *You have to constantly remind yourself of the pain you had, or find that one thing that just bothered you, that dragged you down to do the surgery. You have to keep it fresh for yourself, keep it as close to the front as possible, because if you lose sight of why you had the surgery, it's possible to go back to where you were before.*

So not only was the desperation a prerequisite for the surgery, but the memory of it was also a prerequisite for keeping the weight off after the procedure. Forgetting how bad you felt might put you at risk for finding yourself right back there. Desperation was thus not simply the pathetic, self-loathing emotion none of us wants to be associated with. It was a driving force for both the surgery and the maintenance of a healthy, happy life.

BRANDON: *I will never forget where I was, and I think that's going to be the motivating factor for me.*

The desperation that made these thirty-three people have gastric bypass surgery emanated from essentially four sources; health complications and fear of sudden or early death, depression, the realization that life had become unacceptably restrictive and limited, and concern for their children. There may have been other unconscious motivators for the surgery, but what follows are accounts of the specific reasons they remember as having prompted them to put their foot down and exclaim, "That's enough!" What follows are the details of what finally made our interviewees overcome their fear of surgery, their mistrust of doctors, their denial, their hopelessness, or their lack of faith in the procedure. In almost every case, they remembered the moment in excruciating detail. They were no longer willing to accept a life that felt not worth living.

Do or Die

As already mentioned, the medical conditions that often accompany clinically severe obesity are serious, disabling, and life threatening. But people can be overweight for a long time before these problems set in or are experienced as distressing. Weight gain over a lifetime is usually gradual, although steady, and the infirmities tend to creep up on us insidiously. At first, we may avoid walking because our knees hurt, and then, with time, we start feeling out of breath just going down the office hallway, which is soon accompanied by heart palpitations and profuse perspiration. As one of our interviewees admitted, we may ultimately even find ourselves fantasizing about how convenient a wheelchair or motorized scooter would be. We stop engaging in activities that we once found pleasurable, and our world becomes smaller and smaller. One day it occurs to us that we may actually be dying, slowly. At that point, weight loss surgery may feel like our only choice. This was true of approximately 40 percent of our interviewees. This was their point of desperation.

KARINA: *I used to wake up in the middle of the night and be surprised that I was still alive because I thought I was going to die in my sleep. I re-*

ally thought that I was going to have a massive heart attack and just die in my sleep. I would wake up at 3 AM, and it would be pitch-black. I would look at the closet and think, "Well, I'm still alive." I would even think, "I won't fit in a coffin; they'll have to cremate me if they can fit me in an oven."

At her highest preoperative weight of 445 pounds, Karina's fear was clearly well grounded. That level of obesity is extremely dangerous. At 350 pounds, Daphne's situation was also critical.

DAPHNE: *I had to leave church one time because I thought I was having a heart attack. My husband had taken me to the ER a couple of times because of that. And I could barely breathe. I also had sleep apnea, severe sleep apnea. And my husband himself was suffering from sleep deprivation because of the fact that it kept him up at night, the fact that I stopped my breathing. And he was wondering, "Is she going to take another breath?" He kept wondering, "Is this it? My wife is going to die."*

Mortality was clearly not an abstraction for most of our interviewees. It was a daily and real threat. It was something they thought about all the time, to the point of even wondering about the ways in which their bodies would be disposed of. These are the types of thoughts that many terminally ill people cope with every day. But unlike a patient tragically struck by a deadly cancer, our interviewees had been told all of their lives that it was up to them—that it was within their power to change their circumstances, even now as they faced the possibility of a premature death. Not one of the people we interviewed spoke of their obesity as a random stroke of bad luck. They all "owned" it, and they all realized that somehow they had allowed things to get to that point. They prayed for the will to beat the obesity, not for a miraculous resolution to their problem.

BRANDON: *I figured I probably had maybe two or three months left of actual life. I didn't think that I was going to survive much longer without something done. I had high blood pressure. I had developed something called lymphoedema [swelling as a result of an impaired lymphatic system] of my right leg, which prevented me from working. It actually got so bad that I wasn't able to walk. I was probably in that situation for a good nine or ten months just prior to the surgery. This surgery is something that I said I would never do. Believe it or not. But I got to the situation where I didn't have a choice [525 pounds]. I didn't have any other way of surviving.*

Most people walk around with a sense of tomorrow, with plans for the future. Many of our plans are just ideas about things we would like to experience, even if we are not systematically planning for them in a concrete way. We plan tropical vacations, we plan to get married and have children, we plan careers and maybe even a nice place in which to relocate for our retirement. We have images of the things we have not yet experienced but hope to someday. Well, for a good number of our interviewees, the future had become a picture completely out of focus. Plans were the privilege of those other people—the ones without weight problems, the ones who had no reason to think they would not be around in ten years, barring an unforeseeable tragedy. Our interviewees had a sense of the dreams the weight might be keeping them from, but they dared not wish for these things. Dreaming of future plans was either simply beyond their imagination, or it held only the promise of pain and disappointment.

CHLOE: *Before the surgery, I didn't have a future. It's weird. I knew I was promised that I would be married and I'd have a family. But in my mind's eye, in my human flesh, I couldn't see that happening. I could not see someone ever wanting to be with me for his entire life. I just couldn't, couldn't see that.*

Chloe just could not imagine having the "normal" life she grew up being told she would have. She had a sense of what plans for the future were supposed to look like but believed this could never be her story, not as long as she weighed 300 pounds. At 330 pounds, Lawrence also had trouble imagining having a family.

LAWRENCE: *Why should I have kids when I'm just going to die? Why? To leave them fatherless when they are five years old? I never really shared that with my wife because I always wanted kids. But I was going to deny myself that, because I didn't want to leave kids fatherless.*

For some of our heaviest and most disabled interviewees, the present was all they had. And although we may sometimes think that the present is all we ever have, there is little question that that present is populated with thoughts, fantasies, and dreams about tomorrow. The version of the present in which some of our interviewees were trapped was not the Buddhist ideal of experiencing each moment to its fullest. It was a present filled with dread about the lack of future, with sadness about what would never come to pass.

That sense of being in the process of dying was also about much more than physical death for some people. Some felt themselves fading away emotionally, psychologically, and spiritually. They were losing faith in themselves and, in some cases, in their God. Daphne's story of her moment in the shower when she clenched her fists and yelled at God to show himself by helping her is one example. For some, the decision to have surgery seemed to be a decision to reestablish faith on many levels: faith in themselves that they could do this difficult thing, faith in the doctors, faith in the people whose support they would need, faith that surgery did not breach some agreement with their maker.

ABBY: *I was literally dying. Emotionally, spiritually, physically, I was dying. I could not do anything. And I had to change something, or else I was going to die. I was willing to take out a loan, pay for surgery myself, and decided that I was worth that, because I was dying. But the new insurance company ended up covering it, and so I didn't have to go into debt. But there was a real spiritual thing, too, because here I am deciding to alter my body, and it was such a big decision. Part of my daily prayers were, "This is what I've decided to do. If it's not the right thing, at some point you better stop me, God."*

For Natalie, whose preoperative weight of 225 pounds was low in comparison to our other interviewees, the doubts about whether she had broken some sacred covenant with her God persisted after her weight loss. Perhaps it was a function of her relatively low starting weight. More so than people who weighed twice as much, she continued to wonder if she could have lost the weight without surgical intervention.

NATALIE: *This may sound strange, but, religiously, I'm not really sure that I should have done it. I changed my body when I really was not comfortable doing that, spiritually.*

The deterioration of health was becoming unmanageable for some people. We can convince ourselves for only so long that every successive loss of our well-being is no big deal. When is enough, enough? At some point, if none of our losses matter, we have to start wondering what does.

PENELOPE: *I didn't mind being different until that difference started causing me health problems. It was affecting me on so many levels, in terms of energy and developing Type 2 diabetes meant I had to now monitor my eating habits, which I didn't want to do. I now was more restricted than I ever was in my entire life because I had to check my blood sugar. I was dependent on medication. I had to use a needle. That was the thing that sent me over the edge.*

Penelope had spent a good part of her life telling herself that the accommodations she had to make because of her obesity were no big deal. So what if it was difficult to find clothing that fit, or chairs wide enough for her to sit on? So what if the odd rude person stared at her? So what if she couldn't be active socially? But the diabetes—the needle? That was her line in the sand—she just couldn't bring herself to say "so what?" to that. For Daphne and Helena, other physical symptoms led them to the decision.

DAPHNE: *After my son was born, the chronic fatigue really set in and just got to the point where I would stop at a red light and I'd be falling asleep. I mean, it got to the point where driving was just a hazard.*

HELENA: *I had a lot of weight-associated health problems [at 257 pounds], a lot of female problems. I had a bone-graph surgery on my right ankle done about three years before I had surgery done, and I walked with a limp and I was in constant pain. I would have terrible headaches.*

I would go up a flight of stairs, and by the time I got there I would be out of breath.

In these and other cases, surgery seemed to be the only option. The alternative was becoming increasingly disabled and potentially letting themselves die. That was their point of desperation: surgery or extreme disability with the possibility of death. To some, the threat of a premature death felt imminent—something that could happen any minute. They literally felt they had nothing to lose.

CHLOE: *I was at my last string. I didn't care. I knew I could die. I didn't care. I got on that operating table. I knew the doc had patients who had died. I knew I could be one of those people. I did not care because I was not living before this surgery. I mean, going to work, coming home, going to work, going home, is not living. I was ready to go. I told my friends to just have a celebration because I'll be in heaven with the Lord rejoicing.*

A Life Not Worth Living?

Although most of our interviewees did not feel they were facing imminent death, they all felt that their life had fallen unacceptably short of being full and enjoyable. Some had plans to take themselves out well before their bodies gave up. Life had stopped making sense. That was their point of desperation. If I am this miserable, if I am actually considering killing myself or maybe just wishing that I would die, then what have I got to lose by having the surgery? Others had not reached the point of considering suicide or wishing for death, but were very unhappy and depressed. For them, living life in a constant state of depression was no longer acceptable.

TALIA: *I would put the baby to bed, and I'd sit and watch Lifetime Television, watching movies and sobbing and being very unhappy and eating all the leftovers from dinner and just killing myself. When I went to the doctor to inquire about the surgery, I went because my life felt nonexistent. I was breathing, I was walking around, I was doing what I had to do or*

doing what I could do, and that was it. Nothing more. I had no hope for
anything. I had no hope of ever going back to work; I had no hope of ever
having anything but what I had. It was killing me, and I didn't want to live
like that anymore.

Not even a new baby could keep Talia engaged in life when she weighed 355 pounds. If anything, the baby highlighted all of the things that she could not do. Taking care of business in the most minimal of ways was as much as she could handle. When she had free moments, she would spend them crying and eating, crying for all that her life could not be and eating to comfort herself in the singularly most destructive way. Eating was both her tormentor and her soother. Clearly, Talia was stuck in a self-destructive cycle with no obvious way out. Orianna had stopped taking care of all the little details. Making it to work was all she could manage.

ORIANNA: *I wasn't living . . . all the time at home. I would come home*
from work, I would get in my nightclothes, and I would stay there until it
was time to go to work, on the next Monday morning. Wasn't taking care
of my house, wasn't taking care of myself, wasn't taking care of anything.

This paralysis afflicted many of our interviewees. Sometimes a problem just gets so unmanageable that we freeze for lack of any ideas about how to improve it. We assess, usually inaccurately, that little improvements wouldn't even make a dent in the real problem, so we drop out of the problem solving altogether. The solution seems so remote, so unachievable, that we withdraw from the fight and watch the disaster unfold as if we were watching a movie and not our own lives.

JESSICA: *At just over 500 pounds, I was definitely feeling that my life was*
going on around me and I was sitting in a chair in the middle and things
were going on around me and I could watch but I couldn't participate. I
couldn't do anything.

Some of our interviewees were barely surviving. The thought of actually thriving was a fantasy—it was something other people did. Getting through the day was the biggest accomplishment they could hope for. Some of these lives were clearly portraits of depression.

Depression is generally characterized by both physical and psychological symptoms. Physically, people who are depressed often feel a lack of energy, fatigue, disturbances in sleep patterns (insomnia or oversleeping), decreases in sexual desire, disturbances in appetite (either a lack of hunger or overeating), or a combination of these symptoms. Psychologically and behaviorally, depression is often accompanied by feelings of hopelessness, worthlessness, guilt, apathy, inactivity, and a pervasive lack of joy in doing just about anything. Many people who suffer from depression fail to recognize it or are too paralyzed by it to seek treatment. Depression can also be severe enough for people to seriously contemplate killing themselves, a number of whom succeed in doing so.[17]

Clearly, many of our interviewees were suffering from depression and had stopped enjoying most things that make up full and active lives. Some had even lost joy in the one activity most responsible for their condition: eating. This general inactivity and dampening of the spirit that typify depression are especially problematic because beating depression often requires the very actions depressed people feel incapable of taking. We have to believe that the depression will not last forever and that we can be helped. We then have to take steps to get help. This help can come in the form of antidepressant medication or therapy or a combination of both, or even self-help books on fighting depression (bibliotherapy).[18] So, paradoxically, we need hope, and we need to take action to heal from a condition (depression) that makes us feel that there is no hope and that nothing is worth doing.

QUINCY: *You get used to doing absolutely nothing, really, literally. I mean everything was a chore, no matter what you did; even eating started to become a chore.*

KARINA: *I didn't go places, and I didn't see people, and I didn't parent, and I didn't finish my education, and I guess I just gave up.*

Giving up is a telltale sign of depression. But, clearly, all the individuals we interviewed who were depressed managed to find a crack in that wall of hopelessness. In order to take the steps toward the surgery, which can be a relatively lengthy and trying process, there had to be some ray of light breaking through.

TALIA: *I wanted to save my life because I was just getting deeper. I was be-ing buried deeper and deeper . . . I was just afraid of becoming one of those people that you see on TV that's 700 pounds and can't leave their house. That's how I felt; that's what I felt was happening to me. Yeah, I could go to the store, I could go to the doctor's, I could still drive, but I couldn't go any-where else. I had no life. No social life, no nothing. And my biggest fear was being one of those people you see on TV that they had to tear the damned door down to get them out. And I'd think, "Oh, my gosh, if I got that fat, I'd kill myself. I would. I couldn't do it. I couldn't live like that."*

A couple of women mentioned that the weight had started to rob them of their "real" personalities. They remembered being different. And the per-sons in their memories felt truer to whom they really were than the people they had become. They were not themselves. Getting used to the hopeless-ness and restrictiveness of obesity was turning them into people they did not recognize. Again, this is a common claim made by people suffering from a depression that has not been lifelong. They complain about not being them-selves—that depression is like a thief in the night robbing them of those qualities they recognize as self.

TALIA: *Even when I was relatively heavy but not as heavy as I eventu-ally got, people said I had a wonderful personality. But my personality was shot, and the heavier I got that personality didn't shine anymore because I was so withdrawn from everything.*

We all have a sense of our own personality. We can all describe ourselves as being a certain way relatively constantly, although these descriptions may sometimes differ from the way other people describe us. Most of us have been through short periods in our lives when we did not feel that we were acting or feeling in a way consistent with our usual selves. Many women have a heightened sense of this when they experience mood shifts associated with the hormonal changes of the menstrual cycle, menopause, or even child-birth. In the midst of these hormonal fluctuations, women will often say, "I am not myself." We may cry about things we don't normally cry about or feel irritable or have a hard time enjoying little things. The most salient aspect of these hormonal mood shifts is that when we experience them, we know they don't "make sense." Something is happening that feels outside of our control, outside of our personality. The way women in our study spoke of their personality changes was very similar to that.

> MONA: *I felt like that stupid Special K commercial with the thin person trying to get out of the fat person. And so I think the real reason I had this surgery was because I saw my personality starting to change. Psychologically, I was never a fat person. It would shock me when I would look in the mirror and I would see this huge girl. It shocked me when I would see pictures and see how fat I was because my body image did not match my body, what it was really like. I had this surgery because I was beginning to think like a fat person, and it scared the hell out of me. I didn't want to go to church because I couldn't find anything to wear that looked good. I was finding myself not going out as often because it was too much effort. And that's what scared me into having this surgery, because the minute I felt like my physiological obesity became psychological obesity, I was done for.*

Given the level of preoperative depression and unhappiness many of our interviewees reported, it is not surprising that some of them wanted to die. This wish to die was passive in some folks who just prayed to be taken quietly and painlessly, whereas others had actually started contemplating suicide.

> ERICA: *I viewed myself as a person who would not get old. I was holding on to get my daughter grown. But I figured I would either die early or kill myself before then. I've been suicidal long enough to know that if I didn't have my daughter depending on me I probably wouldn't be alive today.*

> DORIS: *When I did the surgery, thank God my insurance paid for it, and it was like, wham, right now, because God must have known I was on the edge. I was gonna kill myself. I couldn't stand it no more.*

Suicidal wishes are rarely about not wanting to live. They are more commonly about wanting a life we don't have and are convinced we'll never get. And thus, the interviewees for whom suicide was an active thought were all able to overcome these death wishes by envisioning a life-affirming exit from their circumstances. It was a vision that became clear only when the other alternative was nonexistence. It was as if they had to envision their death to be able to see their life. Both came into focus at the same time.

Unacceptable Limitations

Not everyone in our group of interviewees had reached the point of wanting to die. Some of the less overweight ones described relatively active lives. Their joy and happiness had not yet been completely obliterated by the circumstances of their obesity. But everyone reported moments of life-changing insight in which they looked at the details of their existence, at what they had gotten accustomed to, and decided they were no longer acceptable. For some people, this happened at 250 pounds, for others at 525. Our interviewees differed in their tolerance for difficulty and in their threshold for change, much as we all do. One person's rock bottom may be only halfway to the next person's. We all have different breaking points and different indicators about what has gone wrong and what has to be done about it. For our interviewees, those motivating details ranged from difficulties with daily functions to career concerns, relationship problems, and quite simply hating the way they looked.

Some of the moms reported looking around at their houses and seeing only chaos. They felt incapable of accomplishing even the basic household chores. Dinners were takeout or drive-through, laundry was delayed until the kids were rifling through the hamper to see if they could rewear something that was not *too* dirty, and the floors were strewn with toys they physically could not bend over to pick up. Heavy cleaning was out of the question. Only the bare essentials could be accomplished, and even those had to be delegated. The list of bare essentials was shrinking with every passing day.

ABBY: *All I could manage was clean clothes for the kids to wear to school and just enough dishes washed to be able to cook and serve dinner. I resorted to paper plates years ago so I wouldn't have as many dishes to wash, because I was physically incapable of standing at the sink for more than ten minutes at a time.*

KARINA: *I had this little special chair, and I used to do everything in my chair. If I had to go in to the kitchen, it was like, the chair to chop the onions, the chair to make a grilled cheese, the chair to do anything. Everything in the house was delegated because I could do pretty much nothing. I had not been to a grocery store for five years.*

Life from a chair. Not a wheelchair but a kitchen chair. Hard to get much more limited than that, other than through hospitalization.

For some folks, cosmetic self-care seemed beside the point, and, for the heaviest of our interviewees, even personal hygiene had become a physically daunting challenge. These are things that people who aren't heavy don't even think about. They are the automatic, unreflected-upon aspects of daily life. For our interviewees, few activities presurgery seemed easy or automatic.

DAPHNE: *When I wasn't heavy I used to be in the bathroom for an hour, curling my hair and putting my makeup on. My husband loved it when I used to do that. But with the weight gain, it got to the point that we'd go to the store, and he'd say, "Honey, can't you just put some lipstick on?" Why? You know. Lipstick costs five bucks, mascara costs five bucks, blush costs . . . why waste it? I mean, I really thought there was just no beauty left in me.*

Daphne didn't even think it was worth applying lipstick to go out because she thought it was beyond the power of cosmetics to make her look attractive. She felt her weight was such an eyesore that it was almost ridiculous to care about the little primping things most women do such as styling their hair, putting on makeup, or wearing pretty clothes. What was the point? How would anyone see beyond her weight when even she couldn't? But the problems with personal care were even more serious than that.

DAPHNE: *I mean, who would have ever imagined not being able to wipe yourself if you go to the bathroom? Or being able to lean over to tie your tennis shoes? I mean, the fact that you have to buy slip-on shoes because you can't lean over to put them on. That's a terrible feeling. Or you want to take a bath and soak in the tub, but when you have the tub filled with water it doesn't even go to your belly button because you're so heavy.*

Jessica had to get inventive to devise ways to ensure her personal hygiene.

> JESSICA: *I had to come up with ways to clean myself. I would take an old toothbrush that was soft, and after going to the bathroom I would take the toothbrush and wet it, put soap on it, and wash myself back there after going to the toilet. I could wipe myself in the front, but I could never reach my backside, and that was a huge problem. And even just wiping myself in the front I had to do some amazing things—spread my legs, twist my arm around. And going to a public restroom was hard too because sometimes the walls are narrow, and you can't do your gymnastics to get to wipe yourself. I had even gotten this catalog of accoutrements made for people who can't clean and can't wash themselves.*

When Quincy weighed 444 pounds he couldn't shower frequently enough to feel confident about body odor.

> QUINCY: *You would be surprised how many people say big people smell. Well, that's not true. Most big people take more showers than any skinny person because a big person is highly afraid of smelling. The big people I know take two or three showers a day just so they don't smell. They'll change their clothes four or five times a day. I was one of them. I mean, my laundry bill has gone down something fantastic. I had close to two hundred shirts!*

The individuals we interviewed were very brave to provide us with these private, graphic stories about things most of us take for granted. They are important details, because they take the shame away from those struggling secretly with similar circumstances. These are simply some of the many consequences of extreme obesity and some of the details that drove our interviewees over the edge from inaction to the decision to have surgery.

Driving, flying, and going to restaurants, movie theaters, and amusement parks had become increasingly complicated, if not impossible, ventures often wrought with feelings of humiliation. The "safe" world was quickly shrinking. Every venture out of the house held the potential of technical obstacles and, more painfully, embarrassment and heartache.

JESSICA: *I always loved driving, but I had lost my joy of it prior to the surgery because my belly was so embedded in my steering wheel, I could barely turn the steering wheel, and it was uncomfortable to get in and out of my car. . . . I'd also have to pick up the phone and call the restaurant or drive by early to see if the chairs had arms or if there were only booths. I wouldn't be able to sit in a booth, or I might not be able to sit in a chair.*

That's how much time and energy had to be dedicated to even the simplest plans! Making a reservation at a new restaurant entailed asking if they had chairs without arms. And, if Jessica just walked into a diner, she would first have to scope out the chairs before she agreed to be seated. The self-consciousness created by these constant reminders of their weight was a slow torture that could result only in diminished activity.

CHLOE: *I flew Southwest, and I would always try to get the first thirty numbers, because you can choose your seat and you're not the one walking down the aisle to have people look at you like, "Oh, no, the fat lady." You know because you don't fit in the seat. You are squished over. They don't want to be sitting next to you, and they roll their eyes or they make side comments to the person next to them—just loud enough so you know they don't want you there.*

Since Chloe's surgery, certain airlines have instituted policies that require obese individuals to buy two seats. This may make business sense from the perspective of the airline, but it can be experienced only as an indignity by the targeted individual. Furthermore, difficult as it was to travel for all of the reasons Chloe mentions, now obese individuals have to also contend with the fact that it is doubly expensive. How could all of this not be spirit quashing? Even going out to have a good time could easily turn into an embarrassing and painful experience.

DAPHNE: *My aunt and I took my little cousin, who is two years older than my youngest son, to the amusement park. Well, we got on a ride. Well, when the bar came down it cut right into my stomach. And I thought, oh my God, this is too tight. I asked the attendant, "Can you re-set this?" I thought the bar stopped when it hit your body. I didn't know it just automatically closed to a certain level. So they reset it, and it cut back into me again, and I thought, "Oh my God, this is too tight, it's too tight." And I just remember the guy leaning over in the politest way that he possibly could and say, "Uh, ma'am, I'm sorry, but that's where the bar stops. Perhaps you would feel more comfortable not taking the ride." I just remember how I was holding up everybody, and I looked over at the crowd and there was a bunch of people in line, and I thought it would be more humiliating to admit I'm a fat lady and get off the ride than to just hold my breath and go through the ride in pain. So I told him, "No, that's all right. I'm fine." I could barely breathe. I remember being in so much pain, and I couldn't wait for the ride to be over. That was a horrible experience.*

The limitations imposed by obesity can be so overwhelming that some people start fantasizing about what most people dread—ending up wheelchair bound. When that happened to Orianna, she knew that something was terribly, terribly wrong with her life. She was wishing for what strikes terror into the hearts of many people: being confined to a wheelchair. That was the moment when she embraced change.

ORIANNA: *When I realized I was ready to give up walking . . . that was the turning point for me. I saw Richard Simmons on TV, and he was on one of the talk shows and he was picking people out of the audience, and he said to this woman, "What would you do if I told you were fifty pounds away from a wheelchair?" And that clicked for me, because I realized I had been thinking about asking my primary-care doctor how we could go about ordering an electric scooter for me. I found I was jealous of the handicapped kids at work who had their little electric wheelchairs, because they could go from here to there and be back really fast, and they could breathe.*

It's hard to believe that your fantasies can be diminished to the point that being in a wheelchair holds the place in your imagination that taking a trip to the South Pacific did when you were not obese. In a sense, everything is relative. Our fantasies are born of our circumstances, and if our circumstances are dire, our fantasies adapt. Orianna's wheelchair fantasy was a powerful measure of the enormous toll obesity had taken on her life.

Many of our interviewees also believed that their career choices had been severely limited by obesity throughout their lives. For a couple of them, career concerns were central to their decision to finally have the surgery. Brandon had seen his law practice disintegrate before his very eyes.

BRANDON: *Prior to my going on disability status, I had a real busy practice that I lost. I lost or had to give away most of my clients. Couldn't take any new clients.*

Frances had just gone back to school to get a degree in architecture, and she simply could not see how she was going to meet the demands of a difficult college degree in the shape she was in. Until she started the program, Frances had been relatively oblivious to the fact that her obesity had been a limiting factor in her life.

FRANCES: *Within a month of starting school, I knew it was going to be unmanageable for me. And so it was the first time I was forced to confront the role that being morbidly obese was really playing in my life. I had always felt I succeeded in spite of the obesity or that it didn't affect me that much. But in this environment, it was just so competitive, and I just felt so out of place. I mean, I really felt like there was no way I was going to succeed at this . . . All of a sudden I woke up and thought, "I can't live this way anymore." Everybody was so smart, and there was no way I could stand out in that environment. So within a month of starting school I said to myself, "If I don't do something about this weight, I might as well withdraw and just curl up and die." I'm sure there are plenty of obese architects, but I guess for me it was just the realization that I didn't even want to do it. I didn't want to fight. I felt I had to expend so much extra energy establishing relationships with people in class. You are forming study groups with these people, and you're about to go through hell together for years, and I just felt people were looking at me and making judgments based on this package they saw, and it was just too much for me to overcome on top of the intellectual stuff I was being asked to accomplish.*

So Brandon wanted his old law practice back, and Frances wanted to start a new career as an architect. Both had been quite successful in life and had, for a long time, told themselves that the weight was not really that big an impediment. However, the undeniable reality of clinical obesity had ultimately come crashing through the door of their defenses. In response, both assessed that their goals were no longer attainable without an intervention to get rid of the weight.

Issues with romantic relationships also featured prominently in the motivation to have surgery. Some wanted to have the relationships that had eluded them, supposedly because of their weight. Others had had painful breakups, and yet others feared their existing relationships would not survive if they didn't act soon. This included people in stable relationships who wondered how much their partners could tolerate. And even those who were certain their partners would never leave them felt guilty about the increasing caretaking functions their partners were being forced to assume.

> PENELOPE: *Part of the reason I went into the surgery was very emotional* `
> *because it coincided with the longest-term relationship of my life breaking up. I was told, quite frankly, I was too large to make love to. And it's funny, because early into relationships a lot of men I chose to be involved with would say, "Well, can't you lose the weight?" And I'd answer, "Well, you knew what I was when I met you." And when I started this last relationship, I looked him right in the eyes, and I said, "If this is a problem, I want to know right now 'cause I'm not going there." And he hid it from me. And he finally told me the weight was a problem. And boy, did that hurt!*

Even though Penelope had confronted this last boyfriend directly about her weight at the very beginning of their relationship, this had not protected her from yet another romantic rejection. For others, like Erica, the obesity had led her to make bad choices in partners. She knew she did not really desire these men but thought they were the best she could get, given her weight. As a matter of fact, she had felt lucky to interest anyone at all. Changing all that was a central motivating force behind her decision to have the surgery.

> ERICA: *One of the reasons I had the surgery was so that I could have a decent relationship with another decent human being instead of the scum that I'd let into my life.*

Long-term marriages and relationships were also vulnerable to the impact of obesity. No matter how strong the relationship, a number of the married women we interviewed wondered how long their husbands would put up with them. Curiously, there was very little bitterness about this doubt. Most of them understood why their husbands might at some point leave them, as they were no longer the wives they had implicitly promised they would be. They no longer felt attractive, and they were acutely aware of the many ways their weight had burdened their husbands.

ORIANNA: *Before the surgery, my husband's life was going to be, basically, taking care of an invalid wife. He was going to have to be the caretaker. I couldn't see that mental image of us sitting on the rocking chair in our eighties, holding hands.*

VANESSA: *One of the reasons that brought me to surgery was the fact that I was going to lose my husband. I was going to lose my marriage if I didn't do this. I just wasn't attractive. I looked awful and bloated, and I felt terrible. I certainly didn't feel sexy, and he started not to pay that much attention sexually. And my husband is a very sensual man. He always was. And I saw the difference. And I knew it wasn't a question of, oh, we're getting older, or we're getting more used to each other. That's not him—he's very interested in sex—but I really did see a change, a really big change. It gets to the point where you think, I've pushed him enough, and he might leave. He might have said, "I can't do this anymore." I understand because if I were married to a man who weighed 350 or 400 pounds I am not sure how I would feel. Would I want to be sleeping with him? Would I want to be naked with that man? Would I want to go out in public with him? Introduce him to friends and coworkers? I don't think so. I'd like to think I would, but I really don't think so.*

The desire to be attractive had been the major motivator for surgery in the case of a couple of our interviewees. They were tired of feeling homely and self-conscious. They wanted to be nice looking or at least look like other people. For these folks, health concerns were secondary to the cosmetic ones, and they were a little embarrassed to admit it. They were afraid they would be judged as superficial or vain—as if wanting to look good was not sufficiently profound a reason to undergo surgery.

> GABRIELLE: *The single most important thing that motivated me to do the surgery was being unhappy with the way I looked. If I would have said that I had the surgery for medical reasons or something like that, I'd be lying. It was vanity. You're just not happy with yourself and get up every day, and you know you hate the way you look and you hate the way you feel, and you know you've tried everything and nothing works, and so that was it. I mean, it was vanity. I'd like to say it was something else, but that's what it was.*

> LAWRENCE: *Looking back on the reasons to have the surgery, everybody says it was the health problems. Well, I wanted to lose my diabetes, get rid of my sleep apnea. And I knew I was deteriorating, and I knew I would get heart disease and everything else. So I would say health motivated me, but looking back on it, you know there's definitely . . . there's that part of you that just wants to look like everybody else.*

The embarrassment about being motivated by looks is curious given the popularity of elective cosmetic surgery today. The sole purpose of plastic surgery is the enhancement of appearance, yet it seems to have wide popular acceptance. Perhaps, admitting that they wanted the surgery for cosmetic reasons might be difficult for these severely obese individuals because it felt like an admission that looks in fact matter after all—an idea they had spent a lifetime either denying or hating. Having the surgery might feel like a defeat—the equivalent of saying that the mocking world was in some way right all along. That is certainly understandable, but the truth is that physical appearance matters greatly in society—whether or not it should. Wanting to look better was by no means an insignificant reason for the surgery, especially considering the mistreatment of obese individuals for primarily aesthetic reasons.

Doing It for the Children

Most parents will easily tell you that they care more for their children than they care for themselves. For some of our interviewees, it was this primal attachment, this overwhelming love for their children, that snapped them out of their apathy about weight and their resignation to its adverse effects. The realization that their weight was negatively affecting their children was more difficult to rationalize away than any type of health risk or cosmetic concern. The obesity was not just their problem but their children's problem as well. This helped them rally the courage and resources to fix a problem they did not want to leave as a legacy to the most important little people in their lives.

On the most basic level, clinically severe obesity can interfere with the day-to-day caretaking of children, as well the million little things that parents have to teach their kids, from looking after themselves to how to behave in certain situations. It also inhibits parents from being able to actually play and have fun with their kids.

ABBY: *I was physically incapable of getting up out of my chair to discipline my kids. I was physically incapable to teach them things they needed to learn, like brushing their teeth. You know, I didn't have the energy to stand at the sink for twenty minutes to brush teeth with my kids. And showering . . . they didn't know how to wash their hair! They suffered. You know, they would always come over and sit with me. I had this great big recliner so they would sit on the arm of the chair, next to me, and I would put my arm around them, and we'd talk and stuff like that so that they always knew that they were loved, but I couldn't take care of them. I just couldn't take care of them otherwise.*

DAPHNE: *My children were at the most important stage in their lives— toddlers. You know this is their developing stage, this is when I'm supposed to teach them. What happens right now is going to determine who they are going to be. And they would have to come and get me up out of bed every morning. I'd have just enough time to get into that kitchen, pour them a dry bag of cereal, put on some cartoons, put up the baby gates in the hallway and the kitchen. And then I'd have to lie down to go back to sleep because I was suffering from sleep deprivation. They'd wake me up because they were having a problem or they needed something. I would just scream at them, I mean just yell at them all the time.*

Daphne's frustration with her inability to take care of her children was turned on the kids, as is usually the case. They were being screamed at simply for being kids in need of their mother. Daphne just could not do it. Her obesity had severely limited her parenting ability and was now, to boot, making her angry at her children.

JESSICA: *I couldn't push my children on the swings 'cause I couldn't stand up long enough to do it, and when we would go to Chucky Cheese or something, the kids would be in the tubes climbing around, and you know someone would want something or their shoe fell or whatever, and I could never get up to get in there and get it or do anything. I always had to have somebody else do it while I sat and watched. Prior to the surgery I'd call the school from my cell phone and tell the school that I'd be at the front door in five minutes so they could please bring my kids out. I couldn't even walk into the preschool.*

TALIA: *I'd look at my daughter's little face, and she'd say, "Mommy, let's go swing, let's go swing." I couldn't even walk down the hill to where the park was in our apartments. I could get down there, but I could just barely make it back up, and there was no place to sit. I couldn't play with her. I couldn't take care of her.*

Some parents managed to accomplish some version of what they thought they should be doing. They were able to get their kids to sports practices and the like, but their sense of failure was about more abstract aspects of parenting than mere activities. It had to do with pride. They did not want to be the caretakers in the shadows. They wanted to be the parents that kids could show off to their friends. After all, "My mommy is better than your mommy" or "My daddy is stronger than your daddy" is a silly child's refrain that reflects a crucial attachment and brings a politely stifled smile to the face of the championed parent. No parent wants to feel that they are an embarrassment to their children. It is not only damaging to the parent's self-esteem but also painful because the parent can only guess the discomfort and guilt their children feel for being embarrassed.

MAGGIE: *My son didn't bring too many people home, and I went to games because he was into sports—he played soccer and T-ball and whatever else I could find for him to do. So I would keep him active, but I sat in the car—I would not get out and go sit in the stands. First of all, I didn't fit through a lot of things at 485 pounds. He played at certain fields where there were bars. And you don't fit through when you're as wide as you are tall. It's a hard time to get through things or sit on bleachers or sit on the ground and then get up—it just doesn't work. I also didn't want to embarrass him, so I stayed back. I was a single mother, and when I had him, it was at a very low point in my life. I needed something. And I believe in God, and I felt my son was his answer to me. He gave me someone to take care of and to do things with. And then when he came along, it was fine. But I kept growing in size, and so the things that I should have been teaching him and dealing with, I couldn't do. I wanted that to change. I wanted him to be able to bring people home. I wanted him to be proud of his mom. I mean, that's what parents do. You want to be proud of your children, but you also want your children to be proud of you.*

Parenting concerns were not limited to an inability to participate in their children's lives or wanting to be in the front lines of their kid's struggles and successes. Our interviewees also wanted to model healthy behavior and values for their children. They wanted to show them that they were not stuck, that they could change their circumstances if they really wanted to. The decision to have surgery could serve as an example of determination, courage, and will in the face of difficulty. What kind of authority could they have if their kids saw them as incapable of bettering their lives? A good number of our parent interviewees also feared that their weight would haunt their children's futures. They were setting a bad example, and they might one day see the negative results of this in their children when they became adults.

> ERICA: *Doctors told me that my daughter was fat because I was fat. She was wanting to be like me [starts crying]. They said that when I lost the weight, she would lose the weight. So I thought having the surgery, losing the weight, would fix what I'd done to my daughter.*

Almost one year after her surgery, Erica still cried when she told us her doctor's theory about her daughter's weight problem. Not only did Erica have to deal with the guilt of not being able to be an active participant in her daughter's life, but now she was also saddled with the idea, accurate or not, that her weight problem was creating her daughter's weight problem. That was quite the burden. And so a number of parents saw the surgery as a way of teaching their kids to take control and change when change is called for. The surgery and subsequent lifestyle change became lessons in courage and in our ability to change our circumstances even when that seems like the most difficult thing in the world.

> DAPHNE: *I had to take advantage of the fact that I was dying, and I had to be able to use it as a tool to teach my children.*

> MAGGIE: *I think at that age when my son was going from being a child to being an adolescent and getting into some trouble, I did what I did to show him that things could change.*

Concern about the impact of their obesity on their children also took a more anxious and catastrophizing form. All parents have nightmares about some terrible harm befalling their children. It is a common anxiety and a normal part of being a parent, unless it becomes obsessive. The safety of children is a constant concern, and there is hardly a thought more horrifying than one involving our powerlessness to help them if they are in dire need. This common concern was a very real worry for a couple of our interviewees. They were preoccupied by the fear that one day their obesity may put their children in danger, that it may make them incapable of saving their children in a moment of crisis.

RONALD: *One of the things I always thought about was if I was out at the lake and my kids were swimming and they were drowning, I'd probably die before I would be able to help them.*

DAPHNE: *If a tragedy was to happen and I needed to be able to save one of my children, I wasn't physically capable. My children are my heart and soul. And to lose one of them would be to lose a part of myself. My daughter put me to the test, and I wasn't able to immediately attend to her. I was forced to put one child's life in jeopardy to save the life of another, you know. That's not easy. And even though I was able to, overall, accomplish saving both of my children, I almost couldn't save myself. What could have happened was that I saved both my children but that they would have had to watch me die in front of them. That motivated me to take a serious step.*

We have all heard stories about mothers or fathers who find the strength to lift a car or equally heavy object off their trapped children. We have all heard about feats of inexplicable strength or blind courage in the service of love or concern for others. Some of the most severely obese parents we interviewed underwent surgery in the same spirit—for their kids. In this age of rampant individualism and focus on self-needs, we may be neglecting the power of concern for others as a motivator for change. The mantra of change and recovery seems to be one of self-love and self-esteem: "Do it for yourself, not for others." The stories told by these parents suggest that we may want to revisit that particular stance. Concern for the people we love may be a powerful motivating factor, especially when we no longer think that highly of ourselves. It could also be that in some cases, loving others is the shortest route to self-appreciation.

The Unexpected Revolution of Weight Loss

As we have seen, a complex and often interrelated combination of reasons drove our interviewees to decide on gastric bypass surgery. They were all afraid to do it. It took courage even for the ones who were ready to die. Any step toward changing our circumstances involves embracing the unknown and saying good-bye to the familiar. This is difficult no matter how dreary the familiar may at times appear. All were willing to bet that the devil they didn't know might be better than the one they had come to know so well. Some said their journey out of obesity was a matter of necessity; others had simply found the terms of life in their expanding bodies no longer acceptable, not for themselves or for those around them. All chose to pursue a full and active life over death or over disability or over an increasingly stifling existence or over just plain feeling unattractive. But life is complicated, and the surprises on the road out of obesity consisted of a combination of triumphs, defeats, confusion, joy, and anger. Some of it was just as they had imagined preoperatively. Much of it was completely unexpected.

The trajectory from fat to "normal" seemed sufficiently straightforward once the decision to have the surgery had been taken. Everyone expected to become more active, for their health to improve, to be there for their kids, and, if single, maybe to meet someone and start dating again. These seemed to be reasonable expectations and certainly dramatic enough for people whose lives had been so severely curtailed by weight. Well, many of these changes did in fact occur, and people were generally thrilled. However, most people we interviewed described changes far beyond what they had imagined—everyone seemed shocked at the extent of the revolution in their lives and in their selves. Most described it as a rebirth of sorts.

KARINA: *It's an amazing transformation. I feel like I've woken up in somebody else's life. I live in the same house. I have the same kids. I have the same job. But everything is different. . . . It's an adjustment in a lot of ways that I didn't expect.*

There is an old proverb that states something like "Be careful what you wish for." Although this proverb basically implies that within your wishes lie unexpected negative ramifications, it basically gets to the heart of the issue that many of our interviewees faced—the *unplanned consequences of planned change.* They all "knew" what they were doing when they decided on the surgery. There would be an operation that was serious and complex. Presurgery seminars and interviews had detailed the potential complications of the procedure, the continuing need to restrict food intake for the rest of their lives, even the fact that weight loss would not solve all of their problems. These patients all attended a clinic that invests an impressive amount of time and effort into presurgery explanations and evaluations of readiness for surgery. These patients were probably more prepared than most patients at many other clinics across this country at that time. What they did not know was how the dramatic weight loss would impact their individual lives specifically. Most of them told us they were not prepared for the internal, psychological reactions and changes that the weight loss would set in motion. They were quite literally stunned by what happened.

> ABBY: *Thinking about some of the psychological changes I've gone through as I've lost weight—I had no idea. I mean, I did not have a clue that life could be so different. If someone were to have tried to tell me before I had the surgery that there would be so many psychological changes, I just wouldn't have believed them.*

Some expectations were met. Some were not. Some of the things that happened were not even within the realm of expectations. Theirs is a story about the complexity of life and how one change can trigger a cascade of other effects, many of which we would never have predicted. Many of our interviewees had spent a lifetime imagining what life would be like without the excess weight. They had elaborate scripts, detailed fantasies, or sometimes just a vague, general sense of how things would feel. They had figuratively written screenplays for life as a nonobese person. Shortly after the surgery, their imagination was pitted against the reality. The contrast was more life changing than the weight loss itself. There are simply things you can't know until you experience them. Not really. Not entirely. And, sometimes, not at all.

> BRANDON: *It's like jumping out of an airplane.*

CHAPTER 2

Responding to the Kindness of Strangers

Now You Don't See Me, Now You Do

At 500 pounds, I was invisible. Now they see me because I look normal.

—ORIANNA

It seems a cruel irony that at 500 pounds we can feel as if nobody sees us. Yet the experience of feeling invisible seems to be a common one in individuals from stigmatized minorities, as they navigate the world of the dominant majority. Ralph Ellison's seminal novel about racial prejudice in the United States is, after all, called *The Invisible Man,* in reference to the oppressed black protagonist. But how can you possibly be invisible when you are black in a white world or obese in a nonobese world? The complete opposite would seem to make more sense. The sense of invisibility, however, emanates from the experience of being ignored or dismissed. And what do people generally ignore in life? Well, to name a few things, we ignore what doesn't matter to us, maybe what frightens us, sometimes what confuses us, and often what we really want to look at but don't want to be caught looking at. Maybe it's the more polite people who act as if we're not even there, twisted though this concept of courtesy may seem. The more ignorant ones may make fun of us or stare. In any case, when you are extremely obese, being in public can be, paradoxically, a very isolating experience. One of the first things that our interviewees noticed as they lost weight was that people started to see them, to hear them, to notice they were there.

CHLOE: *When you're obese, you're invisible. And all of a sudden you become a person, and people see you. A lot of times I felt like I was saying things to people, but they weren't hearing me. I'd be shouting, "Hello, I need help. Help!" And no one was hearing me. It's like I was in a glass bubble, and people could not hear or see me.*

DAPHNE: *Gosh, when people quit smiling at you, when people don't even want to look at you, or, if they do, they can't look you in the face, you feel very small. Now on many occasions, when I am walking through a building and I make eye contact, the person will smile at me.*

This small gesture from a stranger may not seem all that important to people who have this experience countless times a day. We probably don't even register how often this happens, but our interaction with the world consists primarily of these momentary encounters with total strangers. And these small kindnesses are important because they indicate the following:

1   we belong to a community
2   although we are not close to the vast majority of people in this community, we share some low-level concern, at the very least, for each other's well-being
3   the world is essentially a decent place
4   we are not completely alone, even when surrounded by strangers

Taking the humanness out of these daily encounters eradicates these comforting beliefs and makes for a very lonely and marginalizing experience. Some of our interviewees noticed what they had been missing only after the weight loss—when people actually started acknowledging them.

GABRIELLE: *I never thought I was discriminated against. I never thought people treated me badly until I lost the weight.*

The contrast was a surprise to Gabrielle and many others. Whereas some of our interviewees found it more pleasant to be treated well, others experienced it as a painful realization of how mistreated they had been when they were obese. They had gotten so used to it that it no longer even registered. It was the dramatic weight loss that illuminated the extent of the discrimination they had suffered preoperatively. Most struggled with the meaning of this newfound responsiveness. What did it say about people? What did it say about them?

> MONA: *People looked past me before. I don't know why. I don't even know if I'd call it discrimination. I don't know how at 290 I could have been invisible. But I was.*

Most people enjoyed the new, friendly acknowledgments, but it was not just a simple case of being glad the bad times were over and done with. It made them wonder what had in fact gone on before. Why had they been invisible? Was it discrimination? Was it understandable, forgivable? Would they be able to accept the new friendliness in light of what had transpired before their weight loss?

> KARINA: *I think people are kind of disgusted by you. They don't really know how to react, so they pretend they don't see you, or, you know, maybe they don't.*

> IRMA: *Have you ever gone out and seen somebody with a facial disfiguration so noticeable that you look at it but you don't want to look at it, but then you look again but you don't want the person to see you looking at him again? That's what I now see happened to people who saw me. Is that prejudice, or is it embarrassment or curiosity? What is that? I don't get that anymore, but I think about it.*

These questions point to the complexities of experiencing any major life change, even when it is a generally positive one. Clearly, our interviewees were pleased that they were being treated well, but the change raised some disturbing questions as well—questions that were hard to answer or resolve. Were people trying to be polite when they didn't look at you? Or were they just dismissive because fat people don't matter to them? Could it be that they sincerely did not see you, and you were coming up with some slightly paranoid false explanation about all of this? Very few of our interviewees would answer that question with, "Who cares? I'm being treated well now!" Most of them ruminated over this issue and often asked themselves how they would act once they lost all of their excess weight. Would they too discriminate against people who were heavy, or would their past experience make them more sensitive to the plight of those still stuck in the prison of obesity?

There is perhaps no trait as human as the one that propels us to try to understand how and why things happen. We have a sense that our circumstances (our careers, our relationships, and so on) have coherent reasons for being the way they are, and we are fiercely interested in understanding these reasons. Sometimes, however, it seems that this propensity for understanding causation in our lives is focused primarily on the occurrence of negative things. Millions of people engage in therapies promising to uncover, as it were, the reasons for their unhappy situations. The motivation here is clear. If we can understand the reason something bad happened, then maybe we'll be able to fix it or, at the very least, prevent it from happening again. But even when our unfortunate circumstances seem random, as in the case of a sudden serious illness or an accident, we still wonder, "Why me?" There might not be an answer to that other than "Why not you?" Not too many lottery winners are heard exclaiming, "Why me?"

Curiously, our interviewees felt a pressing need to understand the reasons behind their newfound positive circumstances. They truly wanted to know why people were so nice to them now when they had not been before. The motivation driving their questioning of the positive changes in their lives was very different from that of people who are in distress. Clearly, they did not want to undo the good thing that was happening to them. Why, then, did they feel the need to explain it? We can start to find the answer in the quite varied responses that our interviewees experienced as strangers, coworkers, and potential romantic interests became friendlier and started treating them with a never-before-experienced respect.

Suddenly Waiters Are Smiling

Blanche Dubois's famous line from *A Streetcar Named Desire,* "I have always relied on the kindness of strangers," is truer of most of us than we are aware of or want to admit. Try counting the number of small friendly gestures from total strangers we experience (as well as engage in) in a regular day. These would include smiles from service people, chitchat in an elevator, someone holding the door for us or pressing the open button in an elevator to wait for us, and the like. We would probably be surprised at how many of these events occur, even in big cities where people are supposedly not as friendly. Some of this superficial friendliness is a pure marketing strategy, as in the case of the waitress who says, "Hi, folks, my name is Kelly, and I'm happy to be serving you tonight." Most of it is just spontaneous, intrinsically motivated politeness from people who simply find it more pleasant to act that way. Living as we do in large groups, our very survival is made possible by the kindness of strangers. Without it, our social organization would fall apart. So, most of the time, we take this type of interaction for granted. Not so for our interviewees. They had been denied these common courtesies until they lost weight. They could not take for granted what they had never before experienced or had lost so very long ago.

Some rejoiced at the disappearance of the negative attention that used to follow them around and make them self-conscious.

ABBY: *People don't turn around and stare because I am the biggest person in the room anymore. You don't hear the comments and whispers behind your back.*

JESSICA: *No one watches me anymore. When I would go sit down, people would watch me and wonder, "Oh, God, can she fit?"*

TALIA: *I don't think people gawk at me as much, or little kids don't say, "Mommy, look at that fat lady." I don't get that anymore. People don't notice me in a negative way anymore.*

The situations in which our interviewees most noticed the lifting of their self-consciousness and the dissipation of negative attention was in activities related to food or eating. Most people continue to believe that obesity is strictly related to overeating, so an obese person eating anything at all is often seen as overeating. They are, after all, engaged in the very activity to which most people attribute their obesity. It is something akin to watching a heroin addict shoot up. Unlike the heroin addict, however, the obese person cannot just stop eating. So people who are severely obese often find themselves in a no-win situation. Like everyone else, they have to eat to survive, yet no matter what they are eating at any given point, it is likely to be perceived by others as too much. For most of our interviewees, the fear of this common judgment made any public activity related to food an excruciating experience. Some even developed tricks to protect themselves from public scrutiny when purchasing food or eating in public, like ordering two soft drinks with one large meal at the drive-through. People would then think they were buying for two people. After the weight loss, they finally felt comfortable grocery shopping or eating out, without feeling like they were being judged for eating too much of the wrong thing.

> RONALD: *When I was big I'd go to the grocery store, and I would get the looks—you know, they're seeing this big man filling his cart and thinking, "No wonder he's so big." That doesn't happen anymore.*

> JESSICA: *People would look at what I ordered at restaurants or when I went to the grocery store. I don't know if it's true or not, but I thought I saw them looking in my cart to see what I had in it. You know, I don't get that anymore.*

> TALIA: *If I'm out somewhere and we're eating, they don't look at me like, "God, lady, no wonder you're so fat—look at the way you're eating." And I'm still 250 pounds. But I don't feel self-conscious about being in a restaurant anymore, whereas I felt that everyone was watching me and I wanted to hide but couldn't in a 350-pound frame.*

Ironically, the eating-in-public dilemma became quite the opposite after surgery, as they then became self-conscious about ordering or eating *too little*.

The type of self-consciousness about eating and grocery shopping that our interviewees reported is remarkably similar to that found in anorexia nervosa, and, to a lesser extent, bulimia. Individuals with restrictive eating disorders talk about grocery shopping in the same type of anxiety-ridden terms. They wonder if people are looking in their carts and judging what they are loading up on. They look in other people's carts and are amazed, confused, and even disgusted at what other people are buying. Public eating is also very difficult for them to maneuver, as they suspect people will be judging whether they are eating sufficiently or too much. They often engage in all sorts of tricks to make it appear as if they are eating when they are not (for example, hiding some food items under others or messing up the food on the plate to make it look as if they are eating more than they actually are).[1] All in all, individuals with eating disorders that involve restriction, bingeing, or purging, or a combination thereof, also find food-related public activities daunting ventures holding little joy in store. It seems ironic that those who starve themselves and those who overeat have similar preoccupations, but it makes sense: Both groups are self-conscious about food consumption and about their bodies.

In the case of our clinically severely obese interviewees, it is interesting to ponder whether the people they encountered were really thinking they were eating too much at restaurants and overloading their shopping carts. Maybe they weren't. Maybe our interviewees interpreted people to be thinking such things because of their own self-consciousness and shame. Probably both are true. If totally honest, most people would probably admit to having watched a severely obese person eating. On the other hand, it is also probable that, given the numerous mocking experiences they have undergone in a lifetime, obese individuals might also become a little paranoid and quick to assume judgment even when it isn't happening. Either way, eating or buying food was a loaded activity for our interviewees prior to the weight loss. The general feeling was that any evidence of consumption would be interpreted as being excessive. There was simply no way of eating in public that felt free from the perceived-to-be-judgmental gaze of a public that was probably considering every bite to be one too many. After losing weight, our interviewees felt they had regained their right to eat in public. It no longer carried the shame.

The loss of negative attention was also followed by the gain of positive attention from strangers. They now got the smiles and the chitchat and all of those other tiny but important acknowledgments from the world around them.

ORIANNA: *In restaurants, they used to always put me in the back, in the corner. I used to hate having to walk through a restaurant bumping into people's chairs. Now I get the nice table up front. "Would you like a table or a booth?" They hold the chair. They're nice.*

CHLOE: *I would take my car to the valet, and literally people would hand me the ticket, "Last name, please." No eye contact, no smile. Never speak to me. For years. Then one day after some weight loss, I went to a casino, and the valet smiled and said, "How are you, ma'am? Having a good day?" An actual conversation, an exchange of words! I was dumbfounded. I was no longer invisible.*

HELENA: *At the bank I was always served very quickly, very to the point—here's your hat, and here's your coat, and here's the door, good-bye. Then after my weight loss, I went in and said I had a problem with my account, and the teller insisted I sit down and that they would fix it while I waited. I told her, "You can call me tomorrow or something. You have other customers," and she said, "No, no, no. Sit, sit. The others can wait. You're a customer too." So all of a sudden I am getting this good treatment from total strangers, and it's just amazing.*

Some people did not know quite what to do with this sudden niceness. It was so unfamiliar, so strange, that they were at a loss as to how to interpret it or even how to respond in kind. Strangers had been neglectful at best, and unkind at worst. Niceness had been rare and became suspect. And even if they became convinced that the niceness had no hidden agenda, they did not know how to react. Social skills are largely a function of learning and practice, and, unfortunately, for some of our interviewees there had simply been little practice.

CHLOE: *When people would give me compliments, I would say, "Oh, no," because I never thought people could say nice things about me. I had to learn to say, "Thank you." I used to wonder, "What do they want?"*

Clyde was the only one of our interviewees who experienced no significant change after surgery in terms of the treatment he received from those he encountered in his daily life.

CLYDE: *People haven't treated me differently because I haven't changed me. The person hasn't changed; just the outside has changed. So they've treated me the same way they've always treated me, sometimes good and sometimes bad.*

Now this could be because Clyde was only six months out of surgery and was still quite heavy at 300 pounds. On the other hand, it is always important to remember that not everyone has the same experience. Clyde's explanation is also interesting on another level. Clearly, he felt that his interactions with other people had never been contingent on his appearance but rather on his personality. Since his personality had not changed since the surgery, he did not see why his relationships with people would.

Why had Clyde not been treated badly when he was obese or more nicely after his weight loss? It is possible that Clyde's perception of what went on is accurate, but it is also possible that he is defending against the painful realization that his weight was determining people's reactions to him. Of course, this is impossible to know. It could be that something about Clyde's personality overpowered issues of weight. It could also be that Clyde's gender played a role in all of this. A fair amount of research indicates that women's self-esteem and relationships tend to be much more affected than those of men by questions of physical appearance and obesity.[2] Heavy women seem to be judged much more harshly by society than are men. This is not surprising, considering our general emphasis on the importance of physical attractiveness in women. The fact that 80 percent of obesity patients are women is a powerful testament to that fact. After all, there are just as many obese men as women in North America. One of the men in our study even claimed that his obesity gave him an air of authority and a certain kind of power.

GORDON: *The benefit of being overweight was a desired amount of intimidation and respect. I was Big G. People didn't mess with me because you don't mess with Big G.*

It's harder to imagine a woman saying anything like that, isn't it? Women do not generally get their esteem from intimidation or that particular type of respect. As a matter of fact, women who "throw their weight" around, so to speak, are more often characterized as domineering, harsh, or "bitchy." Perhaps that is why not a single woman among our interviewees reported any gain in social capital by virtue of being overweight. Only the men used the word *big* to refer to their weight; the women used the word *fat*. The latter term is far more derogatory than the former and suggests that obesity may have been more of a burden for our female interviewees, at least in the social arena.

With only a couple of exceptions, our interviewees most definitely felt a change in the way they were treated after they lost weight. As we will later see, many struggled to explain the change in people's behavior and found themselves both confused and distressed to varying degrees by the possible answers. Could something as apparently superficial as extra weight have such a substantial impact on the deeper aspects of existence, such as relationships or, even yet, their own self-concept?

Workplace Changes

Most of us spend a good part of our adult lives at work or study. It is in the workplace, be it an office or a classroom, that we derive a great deal of our sense of worth and self-esteem. Not all cultures across the world place the same emphasis on work that Americans do, but in our Western culture, work is central to the self-definition of many people. Professional success often takes precedence in our list of values, even over family. Unemployment, demotions, and retirement are difficult transitions for many people, and depression is a common consequence of these occupational disturbances. But the sense of self-worth that we derive from the workplace does not just emanate from the type and quality of work we do. It also comes from the relationships we form and maintain in that professional context. Many of us spend as much time or more with coworkers and colleagues than we do with our own families. This makes these relationships, even if they are not that intimate, a very important part of our lives. Did our obese people see changes in the workplace after weight loss? The answer was a resounding yes. As the pounds were shed, opportunities cropped up.

BRANDON: *I've had a lot more job offers since I lost the weight. I've had a lot of calls from other attorneys in the area asking me to do work for them. Before the surgery, that never happened.*

IAN: *It's different around people. It seems like I get more work now that people notice me for me—not because I'm the big guy.*

And this was coming from the guys, who had not experienced the same level of discrimination that the women reported. Clearly, being the "big guy" might not have been anywhere near as benign a moniker as they had thought.

GABRIELLE: *I changed jobs during my weight loss. I actually quit and started my own company. I know positively I would not have had the mental strength to do that when I was heavy. In the world of sales, it's easier to get people to pay attention to you when you are not fat. I mean, I can just tell when I walk into an account the way they treat me compared to the way they used to.*

Again the question arises as to whether the opportunities arose simply because they looked differently or whether their gains in self-esteem made them behave differently. It was most likely a combination of both.

Research has indeed shown that people attribute negative character traits to overweight people without knowing them at all. Overweight people are consistently perceived to be lazy, unintelligent, and sloppy by both children and adults.[3] Furthermore, because being overweight is not considered visually attractive in our culture, obese people often feel they are hidden away in boiler rooms to do their work—away from the public gaze—much as Orianna felt when she was seated at the back of the restaurant, in the corner. Companies do not want an obese person to visually represent them. They are concerned that it sends the wrong message—could putting the obese person up front communicate that the company itself is unattractive, lazy, and unintelligent?

SARAH: *Before the surgery, I was hired as a front-office receptionist. Several months into my employment, the president of the company told the di-*

rector of operations that he wanted someone else out front—that I was not conveying the first impression they wanted people to get of their company, being as big as I was. It had nothing to do with whether I knew what I was doing or was smart enough. It was my appearance he did not want up front. So they put me in the back office, under the guise of being a supervisor, which was a crock to begin with. Several months after the surgery, when I'd lost 80 pounds [down from 308 pounds to 228], I saw the president again, and he could not believe I was the same person. As I got ready to leave the company, I said to him, "Well, am I skinny enough to sit out front now?" He did not know that the director had told me why I was being moved to the back. It made me feel better to be able to finally tell him that I knew what he had said. It took a lot of months and a lot of grief to get there, but I did, and I was able to get that little dig in there before I left.

Sarah's example certainly supports the contention that changes at work were directly related to a change in appearance. However, other folks felt that the changes they experienced in the workplace had come about because they were behaving differently as the weight receded. They had become more pleasant colleagues with whom to interact.

BRANDON: *I've had better relationships at work 'cause I'm not as hostile or angry.*

CHLOE: *People I work with say that I'm more confident, I'm more outgoing, and that I am friendlier. And they tell me that I have this new glow about me and that I'm happy and content. This one colleague told me that before, I never smiled, I was serious, I never had anything good to say. Now every time I see her, she says something positive to me. I feel like my opinion is valued. Like they are more accepting of me. I feel like they respect me more.*

QUINCY: *When I was heavy, if I was to say something to you that hurt your feelings, it wouldn't bother me—it really wouldn't. Now it would bother me because I want you to like me. Before it didn't really matter because I figured 99 percent of the time you wouldn't like me anyway because I was a big person.*

Quincy was clearly engaging in the common defense of rejecting people be-fore they rejected him. This made him feel less vulnerable. He was taking charge by being unkind. That was his way of having some control over the situation. That way, when people were unkind in return, he had an esteem-saving interpretation. They were mean to him because he was mean to them. It had nothing to do with who he really was. It was not a judgment of the "real" him or of his weight. It was a natural reaction to his surliness. But, of course, there is a high price to this way of coping. First, Quincy prejudged people and thus possibly lost out on relationships with folks who may not have rejected him—people with whom he could have had good working relationships or even friendships. Quincy also lived with a worldview that negated the possibility of anything positive in relationships. He assumed no one out there was decent enough to like him for who he was rather than for how much he weighed. That is a hard and lonely way to live.

People are generally nice to people who are also nice in return. If you have been obese and mistreated, it is easy to understand why you might not be the friendliest person yourself, even if you have not taken Quincy's more extreme, generally hostile approach. You do not feel that you live in a friendly, nice world, so why should you be nice? On the other hand, you may be putting off people who would have respected you even with your weight. So we can see how this vicious cycle is created. It becomes difficult to tease apart the effects of the weight on coworkers' attitudes versus the effects of the weight on the personality and mood of the heavy person and the way they treat others.

Generally speaking, however, most of our interviewees experienced great gains in the respect they received from coworkers and bosses.

> RONALD: *My bosses act differently toward me now. There's more respect. I think before they thought my choices were limited and that I was stuck there because of my size. So they would do things that they wouldn't neces-sarily do to other people, and I've seen a big turnaround in that area.*

At the time of the interview, Ronald was almost two years out of surgery and had lost 240 pounds, down from a preoperative weight of 447. He was a security guard, a relatively solitary job that one would think weight wouldn't affect much. Yet, clearly, Ronald felt it had affected the way his superiors related to him, the jobs they assigned to him, and the extent to which they expected him to tolerate these less-than-pleasant assignments.

> LAWRENCE: *In my previous job I was responsible for calling on customers in schools. Before the weight loss, the security guards or principals would always stop me. "What are you doing here? What do you want? Let me see your ID." After I lost the weight, I was never, ever stopped.*

At 330 pounds, Lawrence had been a suspicious character roaming the hallways. At 160 pounds, everyone assumed he was a professional with some legitimate reason for being there.

> BRANDON: *I think other lawyers and judges pay more attention to me now than they ever have before. The weight makes a big difference. I can tell that I didn't get as fair a shake before when I was superheavy. Now it's different. I think there is a stereotype that being thin is being professional. There was definitely discrimination in the workplace, and I don't feel it now.*

It is interesting that Brandon had felt such a dramatic change by the time we interviewed him, because he was still a very heavy man. Only eight months out of surgery, Brandon had lost 90 pounds, down from his preoperative 525 pounds. Yet he was convinced that the descent to 435 pounds had already made a very big difference. This may support the idea that there is no ceiling effect on obesity-related discrimination. There may be no weight after which it doesn't really matter how much heavier you get. Brandon's experience suggests that the heavier you are, the worse you get treated.

For others, it was less about how others treated them than about how they felt about themselves in professional situations.

> FRANCES: *People have not only commented on the change in my appearance but the change in me as a student. In the architecture school environment, I did not want to be noticed. I just wanted to pull a blanket over me in class. But a professor can call someone at random and have a dialogue about a design with you in front of the whole class, bantering back and*

forth. And so eighty people are looking at you. To me, people looking at me meant they were thinking, "Oh my God, she's so fat." I just didn't want to cope with that. I would think are they going to notice that my shirt's too tight, that the buttons are pulling, that I can barely fit into the seat. Are they going to notice I have a candy bar in front of me or whatever? Now it's all changed, and I shake my head. I can't believe I ever let myself live that way. Now I speak up and engage in the banter, and, yes, in front of eighty people!

Frances had weighed 400 pounds when she was sitting in that class terrified of the negative evaluations of her classmates. Dr. Fisher had required that she lose 70 pounds before accepting her as a surgery candidate. A year and a half out of surgery, Frances was 20 pounds away from her goal weight of 150 pounds. With the loss of all that weight, Frances had gained an enormous amount of confidence and was now happy to intellectually spar with her professor and classmates.

So, from gaining respect to being treated as a professional, not being considered a trespasser in the very place where you conduct your business, or fully assuming your professional role with pride, the changes experienced in the workplace were very significant. The gains in respect may be related to the aforementioned fact that people generally don't listen to what obese people have to say. That invisibility and inaudibility issue seemed to be happening in the workplace as much as anywhere else. The generally negative impressions circulating about individuals who are extremely obese render people deaf to their suggestions and concerns.

CHLOE: *I suggested a detailed marketing plan to the CEO of my firm three years ago. They wouldn't implement it. Then they did it this past year, and I said, "Oh, I asked them to do that three years ago." And they said, "That's the first we heard of it." I said it to many people, but they didn't hear me. Is it the timing? Is it the person? Or is it that because you're overweight, people don't hear what you are saying?*

GABRIELLE: *I have the same business associates that I had as a fat person, but now all of a sudden so many people pay attention to what I have*

to say. Like what I have to say is any different now than when I was heavy.
I still know as much as I knew then, and I'm no smarter, no better at my
job, but people just look at you different, they treat you different, they re-
spect you more. It's weird, kind of freaky. It's not fair.

Although most people experienced very positive changes at work, it is, of course, important to note that not all of our interviewees experienced similar gains in the workplace. Losing weight did not have a positive occupational impact for everyone.

ERICA: *I applied for a promotion—felt I had everything they asked for on*
the announcement—but they still hired someone from the outside. I don't
think they'll ever forget that I used to be fat. I still have the job no one else
wants to do. I still feel disregarded, underpaid, and unsuccessful there.

Of course, many people who have never dealt with weight problems feel much as Erica does about their jobs. It is impossible to know whether the reason Erica did not get the promotion had anything at all to do with the fact that she was once heavy. Maybe it did, but maybe it didn't. It could be that Erica was not as qualified as someone else, or it could be that she was overlooked for no good reason at all. This type of thing happens all the time, but Erica was convinced it was all attributable to the ghost of her weight. It had only been eight months since her surgery, and although she had lost 145 pounds, she worried that her coworkers and superiors would never see her any differently.

For some, the workplace pendulum swung all the way from feelings of invisibility and inaudibility to fears that they were starting to intimidate or threaten their colleagues. As they lost weight and started feeling better about themselves, they became more assertive. Some even became quite confrontational. This complicated their work situations. After all, there is some comfort in being powerless, both to the powerless individual and to those around him or her. The comfort when we feel powerless emanates from a sense of helplessness that takes us off the hook from actually having to take action. We know we have no power to take a stand, so we accept everything sent our way without questioning it. There is no dilemma other than our own feelings of unhappiness, which we generally keep to ourselves. The comfort for those around the powerless people is obvious. They can ask anything of us and know that we will not fight it. What we found in this group of people was that the weight loss disrupted that unhappy balance. It had indeed been unhappy, but it was a balance. When the balance was upset, some folks encountered newfound hostility from their coworkers.

CANDACE: *When you're morbidly obese, it doesn't matter if you have a master's or a doctorate or whatever. If you're morbidly obese, it doesn't mean a damned bit. I had a degree, and it didn't matter at work. They looked at what was on the outside. Now that I'm losing weight I think my coworkers are getting threatened. They are used to seeing me at 500 pounds and lifeless. Now I have to catch myself at work and keep my cool because I'm much more confrontational. I think they feel threatened because I have goals now; before I didn't have goals. I didn't compete with any of them. They have been really nasty.*

DAPHNE: *At work there have been pros and cons. My head boss is a little bit jealous of me now where she used to not be, and she nitpicks what I'm doing, but the salesmen seem to want to do more business with me.*

Others put their foot down and refused to be treated in old, demeaning ways.

ERICA: *My boss used to have these "Let's fix Erica" sessions. She even bought me self-help tapes. Now when she tries to have these "Sit down and fix Erica sessions," I'm refusing to. I'm not taking as much shit from her as I used to.*

Yet others found that some colleagues avoided them. People who had once found it comforting to hang out with the self-conscious, self-effacing obese colleague were now nowhere to be found.

FRANCES: *Most of my classmates never spoke to me, especially the males, and now they see this transformation, and responses have been so interesting. Some of the people who had never really spoken to me have been so*

complimentary and positive, while others who talked to me when I was a
nonthreatening blob don't have much to do with me anymore.

One truly unexpected by-product of the weight loss was that some people felt they no longer had to work as hard to keep their jobs or excel in their chosen professions. When they were heavy, they felt a constant threat: If they did not outperform their colleagues, their shortcomings might be attributed to being overweight. They feared they could lose their jobs simply because of the way they looked. They tried to compensate for their looks by working harder and longer hours than everyone else. Although most reported gains in occupational status or functioning after surgery, the weight loss also gave them permission to let up.

CHLOE: *I always felt like I had to work really hard for people to value me. Now it seems as if they just do. I don't have to work as hard now. I kind of coast. They treat me differently, and I think it's their bias against obese people. I do a lot less work, take a lot less time doing things, and I get more response and respect. I used to work from 7 AM to 11 PM just so that if my boss came in and asked for something, I would have it. I had everything in perfect order because I didn't want them writing me up or saying I was not doing my job. Now I don't put in extra hours. I do everything while I'm there.*

This brings up the interesting issue of how sometimes difficult circumstances make people succeed in ways they might not otherwise have succeeded. For some of our interviewees, the weight had made them strive toward greater achievement.

FRANCES: *The irony is that I now feel less compelled to work hard to be so smart because I can get by. The thinner and more attractive a woman is, the more acceptable it is for her to be stupid. That's been the case in my journey at least.*

It is certainly possible that Frances aimed higher professionally because she felt that she could not excel by depending on her romantic appeal or looks. However, even if this is the case, it probably tells us more about Frances's personality than it does about the impact of weight. Not every obese woman reacts to her obesity by overachieving. So what we have is an interaction between the obesity and the specific personality of the person. One person's obesity may lead them to achieve, whereas another person's obesity may lead them to withdraw and not try anything at all. The bottom line is that every individual deals with adversity in different ways. However, it is certainly worth noting that adversity does not always end in impoverished results and may even urge some people to excel. This is the principle of resiliency and a topic of much interest in the field of psychology.[4] What makes some people survive difficulty or even thrive in spite of it, while others crumble under its weight? The answer may be different for different people. For one person, it may be a function of a genetic temperament that is hardy and not very emotionally reactive, whereas for another, it may the support of a loving family.

Receding Weight—Romantic Advances

If there is one set of relationships that we would expect to be greatly impacted by obesity and then weight loss, it would be encounters of a romantic or sexual nature, even fleeting ones. Our interviewees had an abundance of observations and stories about reactions from and reactions to the opposite sex after weight loss (all of our interviewees happened to be heterosexual).[5] It is likely that all of our relationships are in part influenced by our appearance, but probably none more than those with persons of the gender we are attracted to. Our appearance is what potential romantic targets first see and get attracted to or not. Being physically attracted to each other's appearance may not be enough to make for a happy, long-term relationship, but it usually has an awful lot to do with how the relationship got started. And even just walking down the street, any woman will tell you that sexual judgments are being made by many of the men who walk by. Sometimes these consist of brazen verbal comments; sometimes they are simply stares or glances. We had expected our interviewees to experience major changes in the way members of the opposite sex reacted to them; it was their own reactions to this newfound attention that was surprisingly varied and complex. It ranged from delight to confusion, fear, anger, and a profound disappointment in how superficial human nature can be.

Because of women's primary gender role as objects of desire in the sexual arena, they seemed to be the most impacted by weight loss in terms of how the opposite sex reacted to them.[6] After the weight loss, being in the company of men had become a dramatically different experience. Some just drank in the new attention. It was a Cinderella type of experience in which they went from being the unnoticed or even the ugly duckling to being lusted after. This was an experience they had only dreamed of, if they had allowed themselves to do even that.

> ROSE: *I used to get barked at when I walked. I mean, literally, a guy would drive by in a car and bark at me to let me know I was a dog, and now, it's a whistle. And I don't get offended by that. I'm happy that people are noticing that I look good.*

> ABBY: *It's kind of nice to know you are being looked at because people find you attractive and pretty or you have a nice dress on or something . . . I've really enjoyed getting looks from guys. Never had that my whole life.*

Abby was our thinnest interviewee. At 117 pounds two and half years out of surgery, she had truly experienced the contrast. At her heaviest, Abby had weighed 367 pounds. Married and mother to four girls, Abby was delighted that she was being considered desirable even by complete strangers—maybe especially by complete strangers. After all, they weren't just telling you to make you feel good—they didn't even know you. That gave the compliments of strangers a little extra credibility.

This new attention seemed important to most of the women we interviewed, regardless of their marital status. Single, married, or with a brood of children around them, most loved it. Even when in a positive, committed relationship, it's important for most women to know that they remain attractive to other men. You can always tell yourself that your husband is with you now because he loves you rather than because he finds you hot. The validation from strangers is very important to a lot of women, even if we are not active participants in the dating game. It lets us know that our desirability is not limited to those who love us, but that it extends to total strangers who are driven at that moment by nothing deeper than the way we look.

TALIA: *I was at the grocery store with my daughter, and the clerk was talking and getting flirty, and my youngest daughter said, "Mom, he's trying to pick you up. You're getting picked up on more than I am!" And that felt good.*

A couple of the women we interviewed felt they had to hide this new attention from their husbands, for fear that they would get jealous.

ABBY: *For the most part I don't pay much attention to the attention, but every once in a while I notice a guy is looking at me and it's "Cool, cool." It's just one of those things that boosts your ego. One time, one of my husband's friends said, "You are so sexy" when my husband left the room. Of course, I'd never tell my husband, but it lifted my ego something fierce. And he was twenty! I would never act on it because I am married, but it's pretty flattering to have those comments made.*

Others proudly announced the come-ons to their husbands. Part of it was sharing the joy, and part of it was adding spice to their married romance. There is something about knowing other people want your spouse that can make them all the more exciting to you.

DAPHNE: *I called my husband with so much excitement because I had this one guy who was in his car and was young, probably in his twenties, and as I was driving by he took a double look and was doing the "Whoa! Hi baby!" thing. And that just made my boat float. His too!*

Yet the attention also confused some of our women. They didn't know what to do with it. After a lifetime of being ignored or shunned by men, they did not even know how to read the cues. They felt destabilized when men approached them. They had no experience with this type of attention. They either couldn't tell if someone was coming on to them or didn't know how to react if they caught on.

CHLOE: *When I was about 200 pounds [after losing 100] I was at a restaurant with a girlfriend, and when she went to the bathroom, two guys passed my table and came back and started talking to me, "Hi, how's your* *dinner?" and "What are you doing tonight?" etcetera. And I'm thinking,* *these guys are not waiters. Why are they talking to me? And I'm slowly* *sinking in my chair, thinking, "Why are these people talking to me?" My* *girlfriend said they were trying to pick me up. And I said, "How can you* *tell?" See? I was clueless.*

KARINA: *It's hard for me to really know what people mean when they say* *things. I was out one day with a friend, and the waiter was pleasant and* *talking to us, and when he walked away she said, "That guy was hitting on* *you." And I said, "No he wasn't, he was just talking," and she said, "No, he* *was hitting on you." And later he came by and asked me if the ring I was* *wearing was a wedding ring, and when I told him it wasn't, he asked, "So,* *I can take it that you're not married?" My friend was kicking me under the* *table and when he left said, "See, stupid?" My radar is broken.*

For people who have always had more or less normal interactions with the opposite sex, come-ons may seem obvious and reacting to them quite natural. But these are, in part, things we learned starting in adolescence. By the time we are in our thirties, we generally have some practice with this sort of experience. Some are better at it than others, but most people can discern when someone is making an advance, and most people have developed some style of responding to these come-ons depending on their level of interest in pursuing the interaction further. This was not the case for several of our interviewees, particularly those who had been dealing with the social ramifications of their obesity from an early age. Their radar was indeed broken, or it had never been properly calibrated.

CHLOE: *I stopped developing in terms of relationships with the opposite* *sex at about age thirteen or fourteen. Think about it: I was 225 pounds* *in the eighth grade when girls are experimenting with boys. I was never* *involved in conversations about boys because I was not having those expe-* *riences. So basically, as an adult after the weight loss, when relationships* *were a possibility, I thought about them the way a thirteen year old would.* *Physically and professionally, I was in my thirties, but emotionally I was a* *teenager when it came to relational issues.*

Chloe felt that she had to explain this to her dates, as they might not understand her behavior otherwise.

> CHLOE: *I told the first guy I dated, "The only baggage I carry with me is the baggage of no one ever having been interested in me. That's pretty big baggage that you're gonna have to contend with. When you say things to me, you're gonna have to understand that I may not hear it, and it's because no one ever said those things to me."*

Not everyone, however, was delighted with the new romantic attention. The surprise for some people was that it made them angry. It made them wonder how people could be so shallow as to judge others as desirable based on physical appearance alone. It infuriated them to think that 100 pounds ago, they repulsed people who were now attracted to them. You see, women who have never been obese can live under the illusion that men are attracted to them for the whole, complete person they are, including looks, personality, intelligence, sense of humor, and all the rest. For our formerly obese women, that was not a tenable illusion. They had had the personality and the intelligence and the sense of humor, and none of it had mattered because they were fat. Simple as that. This put a whole different spin on the attention they received. They saw it in its primitive simplicity.

> DORIS: *I had lost a lot of weight, about 150 pounds, when I had this one incident that has never left me. I went into a gas station, and I was wearing this black one-piece spandex cat suit with a blazer on top and heels. I was a size 8. I was in a hurry and stopped for gas. The attendant comes out of the station and says, "Well, I'll pump that for you!" And I thought, "Am I in full-serve or what here?" I said, "This is self-serve, right?" And he says, "Oh, we always pump gas for the pretty girls." And I had my employee badge from when I was heavy, and I put it in his face and said, "Would you pump her freakin' gas?" I felt like kicking this guy's ass.*

Would the attendant have offered to pump her gas when she was severely obese? The answer was most likely no, and Doris knew it. This guy would never have left his station when she weighed close to 300 pounds. He might even have been making cruel jokes about her to his buddy inside. This made her angry. Were Doris and other women with similar reactions angry about these discriminations when they were heavy? Maybe they didn't even notice them. After all, if we go to a self-serve and we have to self-serve, there's no surprise there. It would never occur to us to think that someone might have come out to help if we were thinner. On the other hand, there may have been other more noticeable discriminations that the women in our study would not have had the guts to rail against when they were heavy. The weight loss gave them the power to lash out. It is difficult to be assertive when we are either invisible or devalued. It is difficult to fight for the treatment we deserve when we feel we don't have the right to get mad or that our outrage just wouldn't matter to anybody because *we* don't matter to anybody. Frances recounted a similar incident of "going off" on a suitor once her weight had come off.

FRANCES: *A married man in my class who had seen me lose the weight told me that his wife had gained 80 pounds and could I suggest a diet for her. He then said he doubted he would stay married to her, and if he didn't, could he ask me out. I just went off on him. I said, "I can't believe you would even ask me that when you knew me at 400 pounds, and now your wife gains weight and you have the nerve . . ."*

Aside from the fact that this man was already deceiving his wife and thus not making a very good impression, Frances was insulted rather than flattered by his attention. Why? Because the implication was that he was leaving his wife because of her weight gain and that he was interested in Frances only because of her weight loss. That this man had no clue this might be offensive attests to the lack of respect shown to people who are obese. He was relating only to the thinner Frances, and he expected her to be fully willing to join him in the loathing of obese individuals, despite the fact that he knew she had been one only a short time earlier. It did not strike him as strange that he was asking her to essentially disrespect the person she used to be.

Frances had another similar incident that illustrates some men's exclusive focus on physical appearance, and their lack of shame about it.

FRANCES: *I worked with an engineer for a while. We became very good friends and really close, and our relationship advanced to the point at which he said, "You know, I really like you, and I have a lot of fun with you, but I need the woman in my life to be a trophy." He used that word, trophy. I saw him about four months ago at a party, and he came up to me and whispered in my ear that he thought I was a trophy now. He and I didn't speak after that.*

It was hard for some of the women we interviewed to know how to feel after incidents like that. Anger was definitely part of it, but so was flattery. The paradox was laid out as follows: If you embraced the positive attention, you were simultaneously showing approval for the fact that you did not deserve the attention when you were overweight. That's a tough thing to do.

ORIANNA: *When people are nice to me now, I think, "Where were you before?" I enjoy it in a way, and I'm resentful in another way. I don't know how to react. Pissed off or happy?*

It was very important for some of our women to feel sure that the new attention had something to do with their real selves and not just their new exteriors. Some went as far as wanting men who could somehow prove they would have wanted them even when they were heavy. The new attention was flattering, but the *real* fantasy was to have been wanted when they were obese. The real fantasy was to be wanted for who they were and not what they looked like.

LAURA: *Of course I can get men now after I've lost the weight. But I want someone to see* me, *the inside. And I don't believe I've changed one bit from the time I was twenty-one and winning bikini contests until the time I weighed 330 pounds. I was still me. I met a wonderful man at my heaviest, heaviest weight, and it was so important for me to do that because it would have pissed me off to have some great guy come along after I lost the weight, and it's like, "Oh, yeah, now you want me."*

For Laura, getting men with her new smaller body was no accomplishment at all. Big deal. That just meant that you were one of many women they could approach for all the wrong reasons. Frances felt similarly but with a little more rage.

FRANCES: *The very men that I would have repulsed at 400 pounds are now being attentive to me. Earlier in the process I went through this phase where I was very angry, and I didn't want to have anything to do with them. My goal was to find a man who would have wanted me at 400 pounds even though I didn't weigh that anymore. To wave my old pictures at them and ask, "Would you have dated her?" And when I found one who said yes, then that's the one I would go with. Not very realistic, but that's how I felt.*

Realistic or not, that is how a lot of women felt. What's really interesting here is that our female interviewees wanted what all women want: to be wanted and loved for something more than their looks. The difference lies in the fact that some of our interviewees knew for sure that looks were a prime motivator. They now had incontrovertible evidence of how much looks really mattered. Most women who are not heavy probably don't spend as much time thinking about the reasons they are wanted. They may know it has something to do with the way they look, but they also assume it has a lot to do with their inner selves, their personalities, their values, and so forth. Unlike in the case of women who were once severely obese, they don't have the contrast of not having been wanted at all and then seeing all of that change overnight because of a physical adjustment. Not a personality change but a physical change. From one weight to another. Now, considering the popularity of plastic surgery, breast enlargements in particular, one could argue that many nonobese women know that physical appearance is central to romantic attraction. That is why they have these surgeries. However, it is hard to believe that these women experience the same dramatic change in romantic advances as the women in our study did. It is hard to believe that they go from feeling repulsive to feeling wanted. Our formerly obese women probably have an insight into the importance of physical appearance in affairs of the heart that few other women can boast. Maybe this is one of those cases in which ignorance is, if not bliss, certainly more comfortable than knowledge.

A couple of the women in the group had completely unconflicted feelings about the new attention from men. They were not hurt about the fact that men did not want them when they were fat. They even expressed suspicions about men who would have wanted them when they had looked like that.

ROSE: *I would not want someone who would want me fat. I didn't want me fat, so why would I want someone who did?*

Rose does bring up an important issue in all of this. Considering how much self-loathing went on prior to the weight loss, it is partly curious that some of the women who hated themselves so much prior to surgery would have expected someone else to love them. On the other hand, maybe it is not that difficult to understand. Maybe what we all want is someone who loves us more than we love ourselves—someone whose love is unconditional, who tells us we are beautiful even when we don't think we are.

Some women reacted to the new attention with fear and trepidation. Since they had little to no experience with positive attention, they did not know how they would react. They feared themselves as much as they feared the men who were now attending to them. Would they be able to resist? Would they be able to remain faithful to spouses?

DORIS: *When it comes to sex, I'm scared of myself and I'm scared of other people.*

For most couples, being married means committing to monogamy. We usually make a vow that entails having sex exclusively with our spouse. Judging by the common occurrence of affairs, sticking to this deal is clearly problematic for a lot of people.[7] Temptation knocks, and some folks open the door. For most severely obese individuals, the marital restriction on sex with others does not pose much of a challenge. Unlike other married people who may have moments of being secretly appalled that they will never have sex with anybody but their spouses, the severely obese person may feel fortunate to have even one person who is interested in having sex with them. The trick then becomes how to keep them— not how to avoid having an affair. Suddenly, with the weight loss, the horizon expands, and the reality of monogamy is experienced as a challenging commitment rather than as the safety net it was when they were obese. It is important to note, however, that there are severely obese women who feel sexy despite and sometimes *because* of their weight. There are also men who are sexually attracted to big women.

Single women faced different dilemmas. "Gee, how many guys can I interest? Am I supposed to give in the moment anybody desires me? Is it okay to say no to what I was deprived of for so long?"

> CANDACE: *Now it's like, let me see how many guys I can get, and let me see how many are going to be attracted to me. I'm finding it really hard to say no. I feel obligated. I feel like I'm committed to perform whatever it is they want.*

Others remembered their sexual behavior before the obesity had set in and were afraid to return to those patterns. In some cases, the weight had felt like a welcome escape from the confusing world of sexual relations. Being fat had served as a pass out of the chaos of dating and knowing what was okay to do and what was not. These women were afraid to return to the disturbing conflicts of being a "good girl" or a "bad girl."

> LAURA: *I did not know how to say no before I got fat. I didn't know how. I mean, if I said no, they'd do it anyway. I was a whore basically. I know that's horrible. But when I got pregnant with my first baby, I got huge, because in my world a mother can't be a whore. A mother is special. So I stayed fat the whole time. And now I'm so afraid—I don't know what's going to happen to me.*

Whereas some women were afraid that they would become promiscuous with their weight loss and newfound attention, others experienced the complete opposite. The weight loss had significantly curtailed their sexual activity. They told us that when they were heavy, they would sleep with anyone who would have them. They had felt that they did not have the luxury to choose partners, and they felt lucky if it happened at all. Being indiscriminant in their sexual choices seemed to be the only way to get attention and intimacy, even if it was fleeting and meaningless. Losing the weight, and gaining self-esteem, had actually made them much more selective.

ERICA: *Before I lost the weight I was willing to go to a bar, meet a guy, and possibly have sex with him that night, and I'm not willing to do that now. Before, I felt that an easy sexual relationship was all I was going to get. That all men would ever want from me was sex. Because I was fat, that's all they'd ever want from me. But now I'm trying to believe that I deserve an emotional connection too.*

For some, the attention was intrusive and unwanted. Although attention from strangers can be flattering, almost every woman has also experienced it as rude and, at times, even degrading. The fact that a total stranger can feel the right to intrude into our world and make a comment on our desirability can be annoying or offensive. It is not something that women do to men, and when men do it to women, the audacity of the intrusion can be enraging. It assumes power in the man and powerlessness in the woman. It can be an unwelcome, objectifying experience. Some of our interviewees experienced this for the first time and were displeased rather than flattered.

NORMA: *I don't like the attention. I was in a car wash, and some guy just kind of cornered me in my car, and he was telling me stuff like, "Did anyone ever tell you have gorgeous eyes?" And I said, "Back off! Get out of my way!" I was appalled that this guy did this to me, and I did not like it. I am not dealing very well with the positive attention.*

DORIS: *I'm not thriving on the attention. My sister asks me, "Why do you wear that ring? It looks as if you're married!" That's exactly what I want it to look like.*

Clearly, the increased attention from the opposite sex did not translate positively for everyone.

It's one thing to be checked out and admired, but it's another to actually get dates and develop relationships. The latter did not prove any easier for our female interviewees once they had lost the weight than it is for any woman looking for the right long-term relationship.

MONA: *Okay, now I'm thin, I'm out there, man. They're going to be busting my door down. And you know what? I haven't been dating at all, and*

I'm disillusioned. I didn't think it was going to be as hard socially as it was—the competitiveness with the other women . . . all that stuff.

Most nonobese women will tell you that the world of romantic relationships is hard. Perhaps our severely obese women didn't realize this before surgery. Perhaps they thought that it was easy for women who were not struggling with obesity. Perhaps they thought that once the weight was off, everything would fall into place romantically. Although the romantic arena is admittedly more difficult for obese women, some of our interviewees learned, post–weight loss, that the difficulties of dating and finding Mr. Right aren't erased by losing weight. It might have been very difficult to get it right when obese, but it was by no means easy once the pounds came off.

The men in our group did not have as many experiences or stories relating to a change in interactions with the opposite sex. This makes intuitive sense, as men tend to be the initiators of sexual encounters in almost every society. They did not notice major changes in the way women approached them, primarily because women are much less likely to approach a man than vice versa. They did, however, feel more confident about initiating contact with women.

BRANDON: *I can ask someone out now. When I was heavy I would never do it. I wasn't confident, and I would think, "Why would they want to go out with someone like me? If I were in their position, I would not want to go out with someone like me."*

Attention Is a Good Thing . . . Right?

There seems little doubt, then, that most of our folks walked out of their weight into a world that was suddenly noticing and reacting to them. Strangers smiled, coworkers and bosses listened carefully to their ideas, and members of the opposite sex were doing double takes. Only three of our interviewees reported no change in the reactions of others, and two of those were men. The challenge in store for most of them was how to respond to this attention. As we have seen, it was not altogether simple. Although the attention was positive, it left folks with lingering questions about the meaning of it all.

How are we supposed to feel when someone turns to the new, much smaller, us and says something offensive about an obese person? Are we happy that we are no longer the target, or are we upset because that was once us? Maybe both. Our interviewees told us this was a disturbing experience. For some, being let in on the joke about fat people signaled their acceptance into the in-group. They were now members of the nonobese club. They could join in the mocking or simply not object.

> CHLOE: *I was meeting a friend for dinner at a restaurant, and he weighs over 300 pounds. I told the hostess that I was there to meet a friend, and she said, "Oh, is he the very heavy man?" and she put out her arms to make it look like fat was rolling, and I said, "Yes, he's a big guy." That's how people would refer to me. Of course, if I was still heavy, the hostess would have never done that for fear of offending me. But because she perceived me as normal, she felt comfortable calling my friend heavy to me. And I thought, "Oh my gosh, I am not seen as someone who is overweight." And that is the first realization I had that I was normal.*

Chloe took that experience as a sign that she was now part of the in-group and felt relieved. The opposite reaction to this type of incident was to feel personally injured. Instead of dissociating from the obese person, some people still felt that that's who they were.

> FRANCES: *I hear people make statements about other people like, "She's a fat pig," and it just stings me because I still feel like a fat pig, even though I've lost all my weight, and I still feel they are talking about me. People that just meet me don't know what I was like, and they have no clue when they make a comment like that. It still hurts just like it would have had it been hurled at me two years ago. And it's still awful and pervasive. I don't identify with the person hurling the insult. I identify with the object of the insult because I was the object of the insult.*

For most people who have been severely obese, being co-opted into a derogatory comment about an obese person has elements of several emotions, including empathy, anger, and relief: empathy with the obese person, anger at the insensitivity of people who judge others on appearance, and relief that it's no longer them.

> FRANCES: *I've heard comments about other fat people at a restaurant or other places, and I feel two ways about it. I feel honored they are saying it about someone else and that obviously I no longer fit in that category, and I feel physically sick because I know I was that person not very long ago, and actually I still feel largely like that person on the inside. It makes me physically sick because I'm aware that the majority of people feel that obese people are repulsive and that it's the last bastion of prejudice. But on a smaller level, I do kind of chuckle at myself that I can pass.*

For Ursula, having a window into the mistreatment made her struggle to become more tolerant.

> URSULA: *It sensitizes you not to mistreat people because they are fat or because of their race or nationality. It makes you more tolerant of people. I still have moments when I am more judgmental. Sometimes I'll see some-body who is really heavy, and I'll think, "Boy, you need to do something." And then I think, "Wait a minute—that's exactly what people were doing to you."*

The positive attention was also confusing, because it cemented the fact that appearance counts for a lot more than some folks think it should. The fact that the attention had changed from negative to positive was still consistent with the fact that appearance was responsible for all of it. For some people, the insult was not contingent on whether the remark made was positive or negative. The insult was in the fact that people felt free to comment on appearance at all. In a sense, some of our people felt that being flattered by the attention was a sellout. It was the equivalent of thinking the insulting comments had been okay all along.

> GABRIELLE: *The strangest thing is the attention you get as a thin per-son—sometimes it's flattering, and sometimes it's annoying. I was in the mall two days ago with my mother, and this guy just walks by and makes these crude sexual remarks. It's weird to think people think it's okay to do*

that to anybody. I am offended that just because of the way you look, people think they can treat you different—good or bad.

These experiences significantly damaged the view some of our people had about others. One would think that that damage had already been done while our interviewees were obese. After all, they had lived a life full of insults and offensive encounters. How could their view of others actually get worse when they were thin? Well, it could be that they had no idea how different the world would be when they lost the weight. It could be that it was only in the contrast between their pre- and postsurgical experiences that they came to fully realize how cruelly they had been treated before.

FRANCES: *It's kind of interesting how you see people differently because you can see how shallow and transparent they are.*

Feelings of revenge invaded some of our interviewees. They wanted payback. Why should they be nice to all of these people who would have mistreated them when they were fat? And the revenge fantasies were not only aimed at people who had been cruel when they were obese. Some were generalized, especially to men making sexual advances. Some of our women simply assumed that these guys would have treated them badly had they known them before the weight loss. Now they were going to show them who had the power.

CANDACE: *Revenge is the sweetest thing. I find myself trying to collect guys. Just so I can say, "No, screw you."*

DAPHNE: *After my gastric bypass surgery, I had to go have a second surgery because my esophagus had closed up. One of the guys who works with my husband said to him, "Why—did she choke on a ham sandwich?" He was crushed, and I was crushed when he told me. So there's this part of me that just can't wait to see these guys now that I have my looks back. I want to flaunt it, and I want to rub it in. Maybe it is wrong, but when people are cruel you can't help but want to say, "Hey, look at me now."*

The most profound emotion experienced by our interviewees when they were confronted by this newly responsive world was resentment at the way the weight had overshadowed all other aspects of their beings. For the most part, they felt they were the same people. Their perception of *self* had not changed that much, and it was supremely irritating that the world had not cared about that *self* until the shape of their bodies had changed.

ERICA: *When people walk up to me and say, "It's a whole new Erica," I resent that. I say, "No, it's the same old Erica, just less of her."*

URSULA: *It's a real conflict to know that you are more acceptable to the outside world and people want to get to know you. You flip between thinking, "Well, I wasn't good enough for you before, so I don't want you around now," to wanting to embrace the supposedly new you and the new reactions to you.*

REX: *There were some people who chose not to be with me because I was large, and those are the people I would like to seek out and dump or not give them the time of day. There is a little bit of anger there, a little bit of bitterness. But then the better side of me comes out and says, "I'm not going to waste my time on something like that." There is a little bit of resentment there that they couldn't see the inner side of my whole. But on the other hand, I place more value on the relationships that have been in my life throughout, because they wanted me even when I was fat.*

Ultimately, we want validation as whole persons, not as bodies. The new attention our interviewees received could not take away the pain of having once been reacted to as bodies only. It had given them an insight into an uglier side of human nature that most people have an easier time avoiding. Their new smaller bodies may have set the stage for people to become interested in them as whole persons, but their bodies remained the gate by which these people had entered. Most were able to enjoy the new attention and relationships, but they had lived on the other side of that experience. That uncomfortable knowledge would forever play a role in their lives.

CHAPTER 3

Changing the Dynamics
in Your Inner Circle

Your Change Becomes Everybody Else's

I expected my personality to change, but I certainly didn't expect my husband's to change!
—GABRIELLE

We have illustrated the many ways in which the world of strangers and acquaintances started reacting differently to our interviewees after the weight loss. Suddenly, cashiers and waiters were smiling, strangers no longer ignored or stared or mocked them, colleagues started to pay attention to their ideas at work, and the opposite sex was making its attraction felt in restaurants, stores, and car washes. But what was happening closer to home, in the world of intimates? What about significant others, children, siblings, parents, or even close friends? How did these relationships change with the weight loss? Because our close relationships are characterized by more profound and apparently stable connections than those we share with acquaintances and coworkers, we might think that they would be less vulnerable to change as a consequence of something as seemingly cosmetic as weight loss. But that was not the case for the people we interviewed. Some of the biggest postoperative surprises emanated from the inner sanctum of those they held dear.

Everyone's life is characterized by a complex system of relationships.[1] None of us grows up or lives completely alone. But note that we referred to it as a *system* of relationships and not just a list of relationships. The reason is that we are connected to the people in our lives, they are connected to us, and many of them are also connected to each other. By "connected," we mean that we all affect each other—we are indeed *inter*connected. We are influenced and shaped by those around us as much as we shape and influence them. We also have roles in these relational systems, as do our spouses or partners, family, and friends. The system that is each individual's world of intimate relationships is never completely static. There are shifts in closeness and shifts in roles, but there does appear to be a significant amount of resistance to major role changes. We have a tendency to assign functions for ourselves and others, and we pretty much adhere to them, barring a dramatic change in circumstances. We come to expect the people in our lives to fulfill these roles, and they come to expect us to do the same. It's a way of simplifying the inherent complexity in relationships. Maybe we are the people others go to for help, maybe we are the peacemakers, or maybe we are the ones who stir things up. Probably, our roles depend to some extent on what group of people we happen to be with. You may be the assertive one with your friends and the submissive one with your spouse. In any case, most people have a sense of having a defining role within a group, whether they like that role or not.

Haven't most of us lived through the following scenario? We go home after a long absence to have our parents react to us according to a role we don't see ourselves as fulfilling any longer. It is the archetypal "home for the holidays" theme—the reentry into a world that insists on you staying the same, even if you feel that the old role no longer accurately characterizes or emotionally suits you. None of us likes to be stuck in any one role all the time. It negates the fact that we are multifaceted beings, and it makes us feel powerless when others refuse to see our many layers. How these specific roles are created, how we get cast in them, and how we cast others are fascinating issues to ponder. We probably have, in part, acted these roles out, but some have also been imposed on us, whether they reflect who we really are or not. These roles do have sticking power, though, and we generally have a sense of playing a certain part, if you will, in our relational systems. The script may not be completely written out for us, but the general outline of the character we have been cast as is usually pretty clear.

So what happens to the system when one of its members experiences a cataclysmic change? Because of the interrelatedness of our relationships, the likely answer is that the whole system will be affected. If there is an obvious change in our ability or willingness to fulfill an assigned role, it shakes up the roles of those around us. There will probably be a readjustment to the whole relational system. For example, if a woman who has been the family nurturer and caretaker suddenly decides she wants to pursue a career, her husband and children will suddenly have their roles changed too. They will have to do more caretaking and nurturing of themselves and maybe even of her. If the black sheep in the family ends up being a huge professional and financial success, his or her role will change dramatically. Suddenly, the siblings, who maybe took a superior role to this individual in the past, will find the equilibrium upset and not know how to act. The old script no longer works.

The change may be a welcome one in which the system happily reconfigures around new circumstances that are experienced as positive by everyone. On the other hand, the change may inconvenience certain members of the system who were quite happy with the way things were, thank you very much. The interesting thing here is that it is most common for there to be resistance to change in the system, even when the new development is essentially positive. Why? In some cases, for no particular reason other than the simple fact that inertia is easier than movement. Change requires energy, and it's easier not to expend energy than to do so. The resistance even happens when the change spells good things for everyone. Negative circumstances can hold some benefit for some members of the group. It's hard to believe that we can become attached to a bad situation, but we do. Even bad situations can have some benefits—this is what psychologists call "secondary gain."[2] For example, one person's illness may also make their spouse feel needed and secure. Cure the illness, and you may end up with a purposeless and insecure spouse.

Systems are complicated, and it is difficult to predict how change in one part is going to affect the other parts. Simply put, change takes on a life of its own. You can't alter one major aspect of your life without that change having a cascade effect on a number of other parts of your life. Relationships are most likely to experience the upheaval—both in positive and in negative ways. Our interviewees were very surprised by the ways in which their weight loss changed close relationships, in some cases dramatically. It is not intuitive to think that your weight loss is going to have *that* big an impact on anyone but you. You think it's your gastrointestinal system being surgically altered, not your relationships. Yet this procedure can produce such a monumental change in your life that it cannot help but be experienced deeply by your loved ones. It often has the unexpected consequences of changing them as well.

Loving the Loss or Losing the Love?

Clinically severe obesity within a marriage is not an insignificant detail, like whether one person has blond hair and the other brown. Researchers have long believed that the obesity itself may be playing a significant role in many unions.[3] In some cases, the obesity serves to maintain a power balance between the spouses. Each spouse's attempt to control the symptom is viewed as a metaphor for his or her struggle to control the relationship. As long as the nonobese spouse is in charge of "curing" the other and the obese spouse does not lose weight, this power is balanced. In other cases, obesity may serve other protective functions, such as managing or not dealing with issues surrounding intimacy and fidelity. Obesity may serve to mask underlying fears about the marriage being on shaky ground. It may justify a spouse's lack of interest, or it may serve as a reason for not leaving an abusive or unsatisfying spouse.

If any of those dynamics are in place, one would expect some fairly dramatic effects on the relationship when one or both of its members start losing a great deal of weight. Research on the impact of major weight loss on marital relationships has shown mixed results. Some studies have found overall improvements in marriages,[4] whereas others found increased conflict,[5] and yet other studies have reported that some marriages got better while others worsened or ended altogether.[6] Our interviewees provided the richness and detail that make us better understand exactly how this surgery can impact a couple.

Essentially, we saw similar mixed results with our interviewees. Some relationships flourished under the change, others struggled to find a new stability, while yet others crashed and burned in the process of the transformation. Some of the stories behind these differing outcomes tell us a lot about what brings people together, what tears them apart, and how change can illuminate the dynamics at play in any given relationship. It is difficult to make a judgment about which outcomes were positive and which were negative, regardless of whether the relationship survived. Not all relationships were made to last. And some were clearly not sturdy enough to bear the brunt of such a dramatic change in one member of the couple. Although we all root for relationships and marriages to survive, it's hard to argue that the dissolution of unhealthy ones is an altogether negative outcome.

Our interviewees had personal theories to explain why some relationships made it through the changes and others did not. In some cases, it was impossible to know the likelihood that these personal explanations were accurate. In other cases, the reasons seemed pretty obvious. Yet in others, such as Brandon's, there was just a vague sense that the weight loss changed the balance of things, without really knowing why or how.

BRANDON: *I had a girlfriend for many years, but after the surgery we kind of went our separate ways—I don't know why, but it kind of changed our relationship. We are still good friends but no longer romantically involved.*

Did the less heavy Brandon lose interest in her, or did she lose interest in him? He did not know, but felt pretty certain that the breakup was a function, in some measure, of the general change that the weight loss effected. Considering, again, that Brandon was still a large man at the time of the interview (435 pounds after having lost 90), it's hard to imagine that the weight itself had much to do with things. But then again, Brandon's loss of 90 pounds had had a very big effect on him psychologically. This surgery has shown to have an impact on the way people feel about themselves as early as two weeks after the procedure.[7] In Brandon's case, maybe these psychological changes were what led to the fading of his once-romantic relationship.

Although it makes perfect sense that a big change in the appearance of one person in a couple might destabilize the relationship, our interviewees had not expected it to happen. The change they least expected in terms of marriage and romantic relationships was the development of insecurity on the part of their partners and spouses. A number of their partners started to fear the self-esteem gains they witnessed in our interviewees as the weight began to disappear. Their once-heavy, self-effacing wives or husbands started feeling better about themselves. The gains in self-worth were accompanied by increases in gregariousness and assertiveness. All of this was destabilizing and quite scary. Remember, most of these relationships had developed in the context of at least one person being obese. The obesity and all it represented were part of the equation of that relationship. Suddenly, one component was changing, and this change was experienced as threatening by a number of partners.

> HELENA: *My boyfriend started going through an identity crisis of his own when I lost the weight. He had real difficulty with my gaining self-esteem and becoming more outgoing. So he started seeing someone else, and when I found out I broke off with him. But I asked him, "If you were unhappy, why didn't you just leave? Why did you have to go with someone else?" He replied, "To be honest with you, I liked you better when you had no self-esteem and were heavy because I could control you. Now I can't. I liked it when you were home all the time because I knew exactly where you were 'at, who you were with, and what you were doing."*

Helena's boyfriend provided an unusually frank account that was probably true for a good number of partners, although not too many of them admitted it that directly. To own up to the fact that he preferred her when she felt bad about herself was to admit that he felt bad about himself. Helena had gone from weighing 257 to 125 pounds relatively quickly, although we interviewed her almost ten years after the surgery. Most people would assume that her boyfriend would have been quite happy about her weight loss. But that was not the case here. It seems that the obesity was an integral part of Helena's relationship with him. The weight allowed a relatively fragile man to feel powerful. He thought he had a girlfriend with no prospects or opportunities for finding someone else, so he could be sure that she would stay with him and do what he wanted. He did not have to be anybody special for that to happen. He didn't have to be kind or attractive or thoughtful or romantic. He could count on her desperation. That would keep her put and subservient. Most partners who feared being abandoned by their newly attractive and more assertive spouses were not quite as insightful, sad though Helena's boyfriend's insights were. The insecurity simply manifested itself as raw, primal jealousy, and our interviewees were left to figure out the cause and meaning of this new behavior.

GABRIELLE: *My husband has definitely become a different person because of my weight loss—I feel it's all because of my weight loss. I used to be able to do anything before—go out with my friends for a beer, etcetera. Now, he's jealous of everything to the point where I'm trying to make him happy because I don't want to make him jealous. On the one hand, he pays more attention to me, but on the other hand, it's smothering. Even when I have a business trip scheduled, I don't tell him until the last minute because that means it'll be a shorter period of grief. My weight made him feel secure, like no one else would want me anyway.*

It is interesting to ponder whether our interviewees saw their obesity playing this kind of a role in their relationships prior to losing the weight. Did they know when they were heavy that their spouses liked it that way, that it made them feel secure and comfortable? It is hard to know. The surgery causes such a dramatic change that it is difficult to remember exactly how things were before the weight loss. There is a pretty good chance, however, that most people in this situation were unaware of the role obesity was playing in their relationship prior to losing the weight. After all, it would have been pretty harsh to actually think that your partner might be benefiting in some way from your misfortune. No one wants to believe that—not the heavy person and not the threatened spouse or partner. It would not have been a flattering realization for either of them. So it is very likely that weight loss was the factor that really shone a light on the role of obesity in the marital or romantic dynamic.

For Gabrielle, the "personality change" her husband underwent as a function of her surgery was the single most negative surgical outcome, even three and a half years later.

> GABRIELLE: *Your husband's reaction is not something you can control, you know. You aren't trying to cause waves or make life miserable for anybody. You're just trying to do the best you can. I guess my relationship with my husband is the most negative change in my life since my surgery. I hate saying that.*

Although Gabrielle was very forthcoming in her description of her husband's jealousy, she was hardly alone in the experience. Other men and women had similar reports. None of them had seen this coming. They had all been fairly certain that their spouses would welcome a more attractive version of them.

> KARINA: *My husband has become concerned that infidelity might become an issue.*

Only eight months out of surgery, Karina's marriage was starting to flounder. From her heaviest point, she had lost an astounding 250 pounds, and at 195 pounds her new physique was making her husband very nervous. Quincy's twenty-five happy years of marriage did not protect him and his wife from the development of insecurities and jealousy postsurgically.

> QUINCY: *My wife and I always had a very good life together. Our sex life was normal. Twenty-five years of marriage, and we had no complaints about each other. The weight never got between us, but now it's starting to a little. I have become the littler person of the two, and she has it in her mind that I'm looking at other women 'cause she's not good enough for me. I haven't cheated on her, but she says, "You don't love me anymore 'cause I'm fatter than you!"*

Her 444-pound husband was now 260, and in a very short period of time she had become the heavier one in the marriage. Although most of our interviewees had husbands and wives of more or less healthy weight, Quincy's wife was indeed obese, and his weight loss disturbed her. It even put pressure on her to address her own weight when she did not feel ready. The point is that their relationship had developed and matured around both of them being heavy. The change in one of them had a significant impact on the other. The fear of abandonment reared its head after surgery and started to interfere with what had been a placid and fairly stable relationship.

Although the interviews we conducted focused on the experience of those who had lost the weight, it was easy to also empathize with the spouses. How sad it must be to feel, justifiably or not, that the viability of the relationship might depend on weight! Yet how normal and human to wonder if our partner's desire and love for us is based on us being truly special to them and not just that we were the best they could do. It would be very interesting to interview the partners about these issues. It is likely that, in some cases, their spouses' weight loss made them confront some of their own issues of self-esteem and self-worth.

> URSULA: *I think he thought as long as I was heavier, I would never leave him. And I think as I began to lose the weight and people began to comment on it, he became very insecure. He suspected I had an affair with one of our friends. He actually knew I didn't, but it worried him.*

As our interviewees struggled with their changing feelings about themselves, they also had to deal with changes in the way their spouses or partners were feeling and behaving toward them. There were thus three potential fronts that required emotional energy: the individual changes the patient was undergoing, the relationship destabilization, and the spouse's grappling with his or her own personal issues. Interviewees dealing with all three sometimes felt overwhelmed. Most were very surprised that surgery and weight loss could possibly cause this much upheaval. In almost all instances, the negative reactions of spouses had come as a complete surprise.

ABBY: *He is so unsupportive. I thought I would get "Oh, sexy this" and "Oh, baby that." And I can't even get a compliment out of him. I have to ask, "Do I look okay?" "Yeah, you look real nice." Totally not what I expected at all.*

It was especially hard for our female interviewees to understand why their husbands would not be totally thrilled about their newfound attractiveness. After all, many had spent years catching their husbands ogling attractive women. Now they were approximating one of those women and expected some of that ogling to come their way. Some reported that it did, but a surprising number told stories of getting quite the opposite, as far as reinforcement and support.

ABBY: *He criticizes me for taking the easy way out. He cannot fathom the idea that I still worked for it. He just thinks I took the easy way out. And when I tell him that I still have five pounds that I have to lose, I get criticized for thinking too much about my body. So it went from one extreme to the other. The surgery just changed the criticisms from "fat, lazy thing" to "You took the easy way out—what's wrong with you?" I just have to ignore him. I do what I have to do for me and by me.*

One can only surmise that this extreme example of unsupportive behavior on the part of Abby's spouse reflected the same insecurity that was openly described by others. When confronted with their own fears of abandonment, some men chose the route of playing down their wives' emotional gains and physical attractiveness. They probably feared that compliments might go to their wives' heads. If that happened, the wives might start reconsidering the relationship. This "put-down" technique is not unlike that used by abusive spouses who fear their wives or husbands will leave them. The strategy basically consists of wearing down the other's self-esteem and socially isolating him or her so that he or she will continue to feel inferior and less likely to consider the possibility of attaining a better alternative.

Although most of the women in our group went to great lengths to calm their husbands' fears, some of them were in actual fact considering alternatives. Their husbands' fears were being confirmed. Through the weight loss, some wives had found the strength and self-esteem to leave marital situations that they were no longer willing to live with.

> TALIA: *When I made the decision to have the surgery, I also made the decision to leave my husband. I kept begging him to get his act together, but he didn't, and I knew when I had the surgery he would not be there for me. Just like I could no longer put up with the weight, I could no longer put up with him.*

In Talia's case, the decisions to have surgery and to leave her husband were concurrent. As a matter of fact, we interviewed Talia only six months after her surgery, when she had lost 90 of her 355 presurgical pounds and was nowhere near her goal weight. She was clearly aware that her marriage was not working prior to having the surgery. It seems that in her case, the decision to have the surgery was a greater-order decision to change various aspects of her life that were dysfunctional. It was not the weight loss that gave her insight, but it was one of the vehicles by which she had committed to improving her life. Improving her life also meant leaving her husband. Abby came to a similar realization, but only after the surgery.

> ABBY: *My future will not have my husband in it. I spent a life dealing with being fat and with an alcoholic husband. That was going to be the rest of my life. But now that I'm physically able to have a job, to run a household, to raise my kids—now I have the courage to do it. I love him, but I can't deal with it anymore.*

At the time of our interview, Abby had not yet officially left her husband but had decided she was definitely going to. In her case, the surgery and consequent weight loss had given her the feeling of self-efficacy to be able to make that move. Psychologists use the term *self-efficacy* to refer to our feeling of competence in a given area.[8] Abby's self-efficacy for leaving a bad situation and being able to survive and support her four children on her own had clearly increased tremendously with the weight loss. This type of outcome is exactly the one feared by a number of the other spouses who had been driven to jealousy and displays of insecurity. Although one cannot blame Abby for wanting to leave what was clearly an undesirable situation, it does add some validity to the fears of spouses. Not all of the nervous husbands were *that* off-base. Just as these husbands had found the obesity convenient as a means to keep their wives under their control, some of the women may also have been using less-than-ideal husbands only as long as they needed them.

Talia and Abby knew they wanted out and seemed to have few real regrets by the time we met them. Other spouses, however, were actively struggling with the decision of whether to stay together. The main theme, again, was the different perspective afforded by an improved sense of self-worth. Marriages that were based on need were now generating discussions about what the spouses *wanted* rather than what they *needed*. The weight loss and consequent increases in self-esteem had suddenly given some of our interviewees a sense of choice.

> KARINA: *My husband and I are in the process of deciding whether or not we want to stay together. I don't need to be married; I'm not codependent on anyone for physical reasons. When I married him I was in a completely different frame of mind, and my self-esteem was different. He sacrificed a lot. A lot went on that may or may not have occurred had I been a normal weight. So, that's being reanalyzed right now. We're trying to figure that out.*

Karina and her husband were at least having constructive discussions about their relationship. There seemed to be a collaborative attempt to figure out the dynamics of their marriage and its probability of success. This was not a woman leaving an abusive situation, but rather two people who had been through a lot together trying to figure things out. Clearly, she was very cognizant of the fact that her obesity had had a very negative effect on him and that he had stuck with her through it. But she did not want to stay in the marriage out of guilt alone, as she knew this strategy would not work in the long run. All of it was up for discussion. We do not know if her husband felt betrayed by her postsurgical desire to talk about the viability of the marriage or if he was glad they were talking about these issues. The point is, they were talking about the truth, whether that truth was fair or not.

Apart from the more dramatic cases that ended in or seemed at imminent risk for divorce, most couples struggled and coped with the changes. They feared some of the new developments consequent to the weight loss, but they were not ready to call it quits.

JESSICA: *As my self-image has improved, I've lost patience with my husband. I'll jump in a little faster when we are talking. Where I'd have more patience before about what he was saying, it's more irritating to me now.*

In Jessica's case, the interpersonal dynamic with her husband had already clearly changed at eight months postsurgery. She did not experience it as dramatic, but she was concerned about her change of attitude toward him. Attributing her new impatience to her improved self-image, she was clearly saying that the better she felt about herself, the less interested she was in her husband and the more annoying she experienced him to be. This was indeed concerning, considering that it was occurring while Jessica was still a very heavy woman at 270 pounds. She even experienced his attentions as unwelcome. Her husband was not one of those who downplayed her increasing attractiveness. Quite the opposite. He loved it.

JESSICA: *I like the attention I'm getting from other men, yet the attention I'm getting from my husband I don't really much care about. So, there's definitely something going on. I love the male attention. I love the flirting. I just don't want it right now from my husband.*

We do not know whether Jessica's loss of interest in her husband proved to be transitional or whether it ended up deteriorating into a marital crisis. We do know that the surgery and weight loss had effected a very real change in her feelings about him as a romantic partner. Maybe the novelty and headiness of being attractive to other men passed with time and Jessica rediscovered her attraction to her husband. Maybe it went in the other direction.

On a more hopeful note, a good number of the marriages had struggled for years with the changes brought about by the weight loss, and our interviewees felt the relationships were finally reaching a new point of stability. It was sometimes shocking to discover how long that period had been. However, the fact that some couples struggled for a long time and came out with marriages intact is also a testament to their deep commitment to each other.

> URSULA: *My husband does not like smaller women. He likes bigger ones. So we've had a rough three years, and I think we're leveling off now to a point that I think we're better with each other. But it almost ended up in divorce after thirty-two years. It's real hard if you've got someone who does not want to see you change—who was happy with the weight you were. They fight you, and they fight the change.*

This was not a new, unstable marriage. Ursula and her husband had been together for more than thirty years when she had the surgery, yet her weight loss and the cascade of changes that ensued almost broke that marriage up. She was happy to report that they had made it, but she was eloquent in her statement of the central dilemma of change within a larger system. All individuals have the right to change whatever they want about themselves, yet it is crucial to understand that important people in our lives will also be changed by our decisions, like it or not. It is simply a fact of life. However, we can understand how disconcerting it can be for those individuals who had not decided they wanted their lives changed—like Ursula's husband. She was fighting for what she wanted, and he was fighting for what he wanted. We can't blame either of them. On a happy note, they valued their relationship sufficiently to work it out.

As a matter of fact, a number of our interviewees reported that the surgery had empowered them to work on improving their marriages rather than leaving them.

> CHLOE: *My husband and I have had a number of sleepless nights discussing our issues, and I haven't been hopeless or helpless. I haven't wanted to run away. I am able to apologize now and ask him what he needs. Before the weight loss, I would have never done that. I would have run. I would not have believed that I could meet his expectations. Now it's like, "Show me or tell me or help me understand how I can do this more effectively." Now, it's worth the fight.*

Prior to the surgery, Chloe's modus operandi was to give up the minute there was the expression of a problem. Certain in her belief that no one could *really* want her, she was always ready to leave at the first sign of trouble— "Better to leave than to be left" was pretty much her motto. This type of self-defeatism grew directly out of her low self-esteem. She had felt her marriage was always on the brink of breaking up prior to surgery. It had never occurred to her that she could or should fight for it. It had never occurred to her that she had any chance of winning that fight if she engaged in it. As she started to lose weight, her confidence grew, and she started to believe that she could make her marriage work. Running away to avoid rejection was no longer the only option.

A number of other marriages reportedly experienced great improvement with the weight loss. These marriages incorporated the changes, and they thrived under the new circumstances.

> VANESSA: *My husband is more affectionate, more sexually interested, prouder of me. Even though he was never ashamed of me when I was heavy, he's so proud now. It's nice because I see him feel good. I see him look at me when I get undressed, and he says, "Gosh, you look great!" We almost have a running joke about it now. The other day I had gone to the bank and made a withdrawal, and he said, "You look great, absolutely gorgeous." And I had the money in my hand, and I gave him a twenty-dollar bill, and he kept going, and I gave him another. I know he's happy— he's just rejoicing in this because he loves me very much, and I know that I made it very, very hard for him. I really tested him and our marriage, and I think it was very difficult for him to stay with me the way I was, as much as he loved me.*

Vanessa's realization that her obesity had heavily burdened the marriage was shared by one of our male interviewees:

> IAN: *On a scale of 1 to 10, my weight loss affected my wife a 10. She has seen a big change in the way I treat her. I was mean because I was miserable with me. I would come home and take things out on her. She's excited now; she's happy.*

In this case, the improvements in self-esteem led a husband to treat his wife better. When he weighed 330 pounds, he had been aggressive with his wife. Now, at 180 pounds, he had calmed down.

It is worth noting that not a single one of our female interviewees described being aggressive to their husbands when they were obese. As a matter of fact, quite a few of them said that they were much more demanding and assertive *after* the surgery. Perhaps this suggests a potential gender difference in reactions to obesity or low self-esteem. Ian was one of a number of men who reported having been ornery and hostile when they were obese and much gentler when they lost the weight. The presurgical unhappiness of our male interviewees more often manifested itself through anger and hostility than through depression, which seemed the more common reaction of the women. This is not an uncommon finding in the literature on gender differences in the expression of negative affect. Men tend to externalize negative feelings (through anger, hostility, or substance abuse), whereas women tend to internalize negative feelings (through depression, avoidance, or dependence).[9] They may both be having similar doubts about their self-worth, but they express it in almost opposite ways. Judging from this admittedly small sample of people, it is possible that men behaviorally exhibit increases in self-esteem with *decreased* dominance behaviors, whereas women exhibit similar increases in self-esteem with *increased* dominance behaviors. We did not interview enough men to make a valid gender comparison, but the question is an intriguing one. Happy men and women may resemble each other a lot more than do unhappy men and women.

Finally, for some couples, the fact of having to go through the surgery and recovery period deepened the connection between them. It became further evidence of their commitment to each other.

SARAH: *I think the weight loss brought us closer because of all the stuff I had to go through, and he was right there for all of it.*

For Jessica, the final fantasy for her marriage, postsurgery, was "to renew my vows and have another wedding as a thin bride." It is interesting to speculate as to the symbolism behind this wish. Was it simply a question of vanity, to want to be the pretty bride she did not feel she was the first time around, or did it hold more depth? It could be that it illustrated an actual wish to re-start the marriage under her whole new set of circumstances. Maybe both. Her wish to renew her vows clearly signaled a new start and a confirmation that the marriage was something different after the surgery than it had been before. From the accounts of many of our interviewees, it sure seemed that most marriages experienced some reconfiguration. The pattern seemed to hint at the following: Marriages or relationships in which obesity did not serve to maintain the relationship improved postsurgically. Marriages or re-lationships in which the stability of the marital system depended on obesity deteriorated as one member of the couple lost weight.

Is Looking Sexy Being Sexy?

We live in a society obsessed with physical attractiveness and sexiness. Sometimes the obsession is couched in a discourse that appears to be about health. Get fit, eat right, stay young longer. However, the cosmetic surgery boom that we are currently experiencing is evidence that it's not just health we are concerned about, but rather with looking good. Cosmetic surgery is not good for your health, but it can promise to make you look better. It is hard to divorce this emphasis on looks from an emphasis on sex and sexi-ness. Yet there is no perceivable connection between the sexiness of any one person and their satisfaction with their sex life. Regardless of what the ads for beautifying products and services promise, there is no documented cor-relation between physical attractiveness and sexual satisfaction. The young and beautiful are apparently not having better sex than the not-so-young and not-so-hot.

But what about individuals who are severely obese? How was their sex life changed by the dramatic weight loss? The handful of studies that exist on the impact of obesity surgery on sexual function generally suggest positive results.[10] Although there are some reports of decreases in sexual functioning following surgery, increased activity levels, energy, mobility, and self-esteem would be expected to make sex physically more feasible, and generally more desired.[11] There is little question that obesity can interfere with some sexual activity due to sheer mechanics or limited physical endurance for the aerobic or anaerobic activity required during sex. We can also imagine how sex might be impacted by the low self-esteem, depression, and other types of distress that many obese individuals report. So it would seem intuitive to expect a huge improvement with weight loss, considering its impact on physical fitness and emotional well-being.

However, sexuality is quite mysterious. Sexual satisfaction is difficult to connect directly to any one component of sexual activity, including desire, arousal, or orgasmic capacity.[12] For example, in women, there is, curiously, no strong connection between sexual complaints and sexual satisfaction. What that means is that many women who report little sexual desire, or who aren't particularly aroused when they have sex, or who are unpredictably orgasmic will still tell you that they are satisfied with their sexual life. This is particularly likely if other aspects of their relationship are working well. In the case of women, it seems that sexual satisfaction is rated as good if the overall relationship is assessed to be a good one. Paradoxical though this finding might seem, it may just indicate that a hot sex life is not as important to women as a loving relationship.

And so we were particularly interested in the effect that the surgery and consequent weight loss would have on the sex lives of the women we interviewed. Although it might seem obvious to predict that sex will improve when we feel better about the way we look and about ourselves in general, we expected that the story might be more complicated than that. And it was. As far the mechanics of sexual intercourse and its various positions, the consensus seemed to be that everything was easier to accomplish. But, again, satisfying sex is about a lot more than having the stamina or being able to contort oneself into a specific position.

It is no surprise that some of the women who had decided at the time of surgery or shortly thereafter to leave their marriages reported no improvements in sexual desire or satisfaction after surgery. They probably did not have fulfilling sexual lives before, and the surgery had done nothing to improve their relationships. If anything, the surgery and weight loss had illuminated the deficits of these marriages. These women did not tie their lack of desire to the weight loss.

ABBY: *As far as sex itself, it's easier. It is physically more fulfilling. Do I desire it? Not at all. But that doesn't have anything to do with the weight loss—it just has to do with the way I feel about him.*

A good number of our interviewees in happy marriages or who were single prior to surgery reported very real gains after the weight loss.

SARAH: *Our sexual life has improved since I lost the weight. I don't know if it was the physical largeness which mechanically prevented sex from happening before or whether it was the physical appearance insofar as my husband probably didn't find me attractive and I didn't find myself attractive. But it's back.*

REX: *Losing the weight opened up a lot of opportunities in terms of sexual activity. The desire had always been there, but now it's physically easier to get things done different ways.*

These couples seemed to chalk up the improvements to their newfound ability to move around and diversify their sexual activity, as well as to gains in physical attractiveness. Other couples attributed the improvements in their sex lives to the fact that they were simply getting along a lot better.

GORDON: *Our sex life is better, we are more romantic, but it's because we have more tolerance for stupid things.*

Gordon and his wife had stopped arguing about little things once he lost weight. This had resulted in an enhanced sense of closeness and passion. For those with more alternative forms of sexual expression, the weight loss had allowed them to rediscover pleasure in activities that they had come to abandon because of their weight.

PENELOPE: *My sexual desire has not changed because that has always been such a mental thing for me, but now I can actually enjoy a lot of the BDSM [bondage, discipline, sadomasochism] things like spanking and bondage which I had lost pleasure in when I was very heavy.*

It may be shocking for some people to read that Penelope had a penchant for a sexual activity that many people would find exotic or even scary, but it is a good reminder to all of us that severely obese people can be just as sexual and adventurous as anybody else, if not more so.

A decrease in sexual desire was the most common and the most unexpected report of postsurgical sexual outcomes in our group. The majority of the women we interviewed told us that, much to their surprise, their sexual desire had decreased after surgery—and these were not women in troubled marriages. They did report that sex was easier, that once they were engaged in the activity they became aroused, but they had lost all spontaneous desire for it. Most didn't understand why.

DAPHNE: *I seem to have lost part of my desire for sexual intercourse. Even though sexual intercourse is always a pleasure, I just don't seem to get in the mood on my own. Making love itself is a lot better now, and more pleasurable for me, as well as my spouse, but I rarely want it.*

For Jessica, the loss of desire was even starting to feel like full-on aversion.

JESSICA: *I've lost all sexual desire. I don't have any, I couldn't care less about it, and I know that bothers my husband very badly. When he talks about anything sexual, I get a weird feeling inside. It's not just that my head doesn't want it; my actual body cringes, like something's disgusting or something. I absolutely love him to death—he's a wonderful man, worships the ground I walk on, and he's a great father. I just have to get over this sex thing with him.*

Most women who reported this loss of sexual desire did not know why it was happening, but a couple of them attributed it directly to their appearance. Their appearance? Didn't they look better now that they had lost all that weight? Well, one of the consequences of losing a great deal of weight is that you are left with a lot of excess skin. One of our interviewees even described having to tuck the extra sagging skin into his pants, as you would a shirt. You can have a number of surgeries to correct the sagginess.[13] The most common ones are the abdominoplasty and the panniculectomy, which are surgeries designed to remove the excess fat and skin left after being severely obese and then losing massive amounts of weight. Unlike the panniculectomy, the abdominoplasty also tightens abdominal muscles. Other not as common procedures are body, breast, arm, and thigh lifts. Without one or more of these cosmetic surgeries, many interviewees felt that the weight loss had not resulted in a more attractive naked them. All dressed up they looked great, but naked they did not feel attractive. Some women reported having felt much sexier in the nude when they were heavy than after the surgery.

> ORIANNA: *The biggest negative effect of the surgery has been on our sex life or lack of it. I don't want anything to do with it. It's not that I felt sexy in my fat body, but my husband loved me this and that way, and it was okay. Yeah, I'd glance in the mirror and see the big old ass going by, but it was okay. Now, all I see is what hangs and what sags, and when we are having those intimate moments, all I can think of is where my boobs are, what's hanging there, and oh my God, how can he? I'm not thinking about the sensation or the feelings of pleasure but just that there are folds and folds and wrinkles and wrinkles, and how can he look at that? I hate that. He says it's okay for him, but to me it's not okay. I want reconstructive surgery very badly. He's against it.*

The expense of these reconstructive surgeries is not typically covered by insurance, unless there is proof that the excess skin impairs one's functioning or causes chaffing and rashes. The surgeries can be too expensive for most patients to pay out-of-pocket. Some of our heaviest interviewees, however, felt pretty strongly that these were not optional procedures—that the cosmetic result of massive weight loss without them was simply unacceptable.

Apart from the very understandable interference of sagging skin, do we have any reason to believe that this surgery should result in a decrease in sexual desire? It is hard to know, but there are some physiological changes that could conceivably produce lower levels of desire. For example, estrogen levels do decrease with dramatic weight loss, and this could potentially be physiologically linked to a decrease in sexual desire.[14] Although estrogen does not have a very strong direct link to sexual desire, estrogen is needed for the production of testosterone, and the link between testosterone and sexual desire is indeed a stronger one.[15] On the other hand, the reasons could also be psychological or relational. It could be that with the weight loss and increases in self-esteem, women started finding their partners less desirable. It could also be that with the increase in sexual advances from strangers and acquaintances, their sexual fantasies were drawn away from established relationships. It may even be the case that with the increase in self-worth, these women needed less reinforcement about their desirability, a reinforcement previously obtained from sexual intimacy. Any one or combination of these factors could conceivably have contributed to a decrease in sexual desire for their presurgical partner. Sexual desire is a complex phenomenon that cannot be easily predicted by weight loss or gain.

Perhaps the most important lesson to be derived from the mixed outcomes in terms of sexuality is that we can assume very little about the way in which weight loss will impact lives. What seems obvious is often not obvious at all. To most people it would seem obvious that weight loss would improve sexual lives. Yet that was not the case for a number of our interviewees. *Sexual* is perhaps the last word we would associate with the clinically severely obese, yet a significant number of the women in our study felt more sexual before the surgery—before their dramatic weight loss. So much for our mass media–influenced ideas about sexiness as indelibly linked to thinness!

From the Mouths of Babes

Although the surgery might have had an unexpected and unintended effect on marital and romantic relationships, its effect on our interviewees' relationships with their children was most definitely hoped for and intended. Almost every parent in our group listed concern for their children as a primary motivation for having the surgery. Parents seemed acutely aware of the impact their obesity might be having on their kids. They worried about these relationships on a number of levels. At the most basic level, parents feared that they were setting a bad example, that they were modeling for their kids an unhealthy and hopeless lifestyle. There were also concerns about physically not being able to teach their kids the simple activities of daily living, play with them, or join them in their sports and other pursuits. At the most poignant levels, parents did not want their kids to be embarrassed by them. They also feared that their physical disability might one day result in their inability to save their children's lives were some catastrophe to strike.

And, indeed, changes in relationships with kids were perhaps the most dramatic and consistent of all the changes reported. Quite suddenly, patients were able to become involved in the daily type of lessons that most parents take for granted. There was clearly a lot of catching up to do.

> ABBY: *After the weight loss, I had to take my ten-year-old daughter in the shower and say, "This is how much shampoo you have to use. Now we have to make sure that you know how to rinse your hair." I had to teach her how to wash her body. So I've had to backtrack a lot and teach them. They didn't know how to pick up their clothes.*

For all the press that obesity and gastric bypass surgery get these days, it is rare to read anything about the impact of severe obesity on parenting. We could not find a single reference in the research literature regarding the impact of this type of surgery on the children of patients. Yet hearing descriptions such as Abby's demonstrates how vital a parent's mobility and health are to the rearing of children. With difficulty moving around and with little energy, Abby had lapsed in many of her parenting responsibilities. Her ten year old did not know how to wash her hair, so she was probably going to school with dirty hair. Maybe she was being teased for this. The teasing may have started creating in Abby's little girl feelings of low self-esteem that could start a pattern of social isolation that might haunt her for a lifetime. We do not know if this happened or if it would have had Abby not had the surgery. It is plausible, however, and it highlights how a failure of parenting even at this micro a level can have a huge impact on a child's life and possibly on his or her future. It is a perfect illustration of systems theory—how something happening at one level of the system can have a huge effect on another. In Abby's case, she was conscious of the potential impact, and she experienced anguish at her failure. But some of the parents in our study had not fully realized how their weight and weight-related conditions were affecting their children. Our conversations with them led us to believe that, even though some had surgery primarily to improve conditions for their children, they were surprised at how wide-ranging and positive its effect on the children actually turned out to be.

Our interviewees' kids became healthier as they saw at least one parent model healthy behavior. Some parents purposely became actively involved in ensuring that their children did not follow in their path to obesity. They became committed to helping their kids manage what might be a genetic vulnerability to gain weight. The surgery had taught them that a genetic propensity need not be experienced as a life-or-death sentence, but, rather, it can serve as a reminder that special attention may need to be exerted to control for certain tendencies. That is a far cry from the determinism that many of our patients felt prior to the surgery, when they were in no position to teach their kids health lessons. How could they, when they themselves were setting an example contrary to the lesson? The parents had to make their own changes before attempting to communicate effectively with their kids about obesity and health.

IAN: *I'm teaching my kids a different way of eating.*

RONALD: *My children got involved in caring for me after the surgery, and it has also made them more health conscious.*

ABBY: *My second daughter reads labels now, and she can tell you how many calories and how many grams of fat the food has. It's really fun! I spent a lifetime suffering, and I don't want to see my girls go through that. My daughter came home one day crying because someone had teased her, and it broke my heart. So I had her watch the* Oprah *show on overweight kids, and I watched it with her. "See, we can do these things," I told her.*

Abby could hardly have made this point with her daughter if she was still stuck in the obesity trap. The power of "we" was born in part of the surgery and its consequent dietary regimen.

But parenting is about so much more than directives about brushing teeth and picking up clothes or eating right. It is also about fun. It's about doing things together and laughing and enjoying life. Our interviewees noticed a huge difference in their ability to participate in these activities and in the consequent joy their active presence brought to their kids' lives.

DAPHNE: *I can do things I want to do with my kids. I mean, I've sat on the floor with my son just two weeks ago and played cars on this little racetrack.*

MAGGIE: *When I lost the weight it was a very positive thing for my son because I was able to go to the games and participate and yell and scream and even get kicked out for saying derogatory things to the referee!*

ABBY: *We go out, and we walk, or we run, or I even got on their bike and rode their bike down the street, and they were shocked that I could ride a bike! We talk. I read them stories now. Because I am not depressed, just talking to them is different. I think that they understand more that I care about them because I talk to them more.*

KARINA: *The other night we went to the diner and listened to fifties music, and it was fun, and I couldn't remember the last time I had gone out to dinner with my kids.*

One of the most moving manifestations of the change in the relationship between parents and children after surgery had to do with the joy children felt when they saw their parents happy. All too often, parents fall into the trap of thinking that as long as they are providing for their kids and treating them right, they are doing their job. But kids need more than that. They yearn to see their parents laugh and enjoy life and be content, arguably as much as parents want to witness that in their kids. Yet we often underestimate how much our own personal happiness means to our children, how much it affects them, how much they need for us to be okay. Our being okay means they're going to be okay. Our being miserable or depressed instills an empathic sadness in them; it makes them wonder if they are the cause of our unhappiness, and it makes them attempt to compensate for our lack of happiness. It instills doubts about the security of their home and well-being. And that is no way to grow up.

> KARINA: *I had no idea how much of an impact my losing weight had on my thirteen-year-old son. It had been his job to unload the dishwasher, and one day he came home and I was unloading it. Suddenly, without having looked behind me, I sensed him just standing there looking at me. And I said, "What's the matter, are you sick?" And he said, "No, you're doing the dishes." To which I replied, "I know, but you were late and enjoying yourself, and I thought I'd just do them." And he said, "No, I mean look at you—you're doing the dishes." He was so pleased that I could stand there and do it. It was a great moment for him.*

> TALIA: *My son and his wife took me out to a funny show. At one point I was laughing so hard, and I turned around and saw that my son had started crying. He hugged me and said, "Mom, I've never seen you so happy."*

Karina's thirteen year old and Talia's adult son expressed in powerful ways how much their mothers' weight loss had affected them. It had made their moms active and happy, which in turn made them happy. Both of these gestures—the standing there in shock and the crying—speak volumes about how hard it had been for these kids to see their parents suffer. For our interviewees, these expressions of joy from their sons and daughters seemed to come as a surprise, and it meant the world to them. What better reinforcement for our efforts than the smile on our child's face? Children continued to serve as an important source of support through the difficulties of dieting and major life changes following the surgery. They were daily living proof that it was all worth it.

> ABBY: *My children are my biggest support. They always say, "Mommy, you are so pretty."*

> MAGGIE: *My son is totally on top of everything I eat and whether I am following the right regimen. He does scientific studies on me. He has gone to the doctor with me to go through all the blood work. He'll call me and*

say, "What did you eat today? How many times did you throw up? Did you take your pills?" We fight like cats and dogs, but we are very close, and he monitors me.

Perhaps the most profound impact that the surgery had on our interviewees' children was in providing them with an example of courage and determination. Their parents were not just going to accept a life-threatening disability lying down. They were going to show their kids that positive change is not only possible but also worth the sacrifices it can entail. A number of our interviewees felt strongly that their surgery had had that kind of deep impact on their children.

MAGGIE: *I had the surgery when my son was in that transition from being a boy to an adolescent, and I did what I did to show him that things could change. I think it changed him as well. I changed in one way, and he changed in another. He became more positive and found that he could change his life too. We talk about breaking the mold. Children carry the baggage from their parents, but at some point you are old enough to become what you want. Society doesn't teach you that. My son is now in his second year of medical school, and he plans to become a surgeon. It's very possible that my going through the surgery had a lot to do with that.*

And thus the change of the moms and dads had become the change of the children.

Rocking the Friendship Boat

Friends are an important part of our lives. They can be our second family, and they can also contribute to our lives in unique ways that families can't or don't. They can be a key source of support, a reality test when we're not sure of our own thoughts or reactions. They are companions in both sadness and joy, and a welcome temporary escape from families when we need to be around people whose demands on us are altogether different and usually lighter. We cry with them, and we laugh with them. Different people express different levels of need when it comes to having friends in their lives, but most people will tell you that friends are important.

For this reason, we were interested in the extent to which gastric bypass surgery had impacted these relationships. We collected a wealth of information ranging from good to bad to medium outcomes, but few interviewees had difficulty summoning up how their friendships had been impacted. A couple of folks rejected the notion out-of-hand that weight loss would have impacted their friendships.

FRANCES: *The small network of people I considered my friends at 400 pounds are all still there.*

SARAH: *I still have the same group of friends I had when I was heavy, but that's because I'm the same person I was when I was 308 pounds.*

CLYDE: *My friends are still my friends. We all treat each other the same.*

The vast majority, however, did not respond with, "Why would my friendships be impacted by my weight loss?" We had suspected this would be an important question, and the richness of the responses we heard confirmed our suspicions.

A number of people reported very real gains in their friendships after weight loss and attributed it mostly to their increased level of activity. No longer isolated in their homes, they could now join in the world of outings and get-togethers.

BRANDON: *I've got some friends who have invited me to different places, and before I would never have taken them up on it, but now I do. I am closer to my friends now because I spend more time with them because I want to go out. Going out with friends no longer means worrying about whether I am going to fit into chairs at the restaurant. That has brought us closer together.*

Others boasted that their friends had been tremendously supportive through the surgery and the months and years of consequent weight loss. It was clear from their responses that this support had played a very important role in their recovery and continued efforts to lose weight.

JESSICA: *My friends have been very, very supportive. They always tell me I look beautiful.*

ROSE: *My friends are delighted that I'm thin. They ask me to go into their closets and borrow their clothes. Not one of them rejected me for getting thin.*

This may seem like the natural thing for friends to do, but being supportive of a buddy who has set a goal for weight loss or for any other accomplishment can be a tricky affair. We want to communicate our encouragement and reinforcement of their aspirations, but we also need to communicate that our love and respect for them are not contingent on their achieving specific goals. We want to support them in their efforts while letting them know that we will love them or, at least, not judge them if they don't succeed. That is quite the tightrope to walk: to express unconditional love while encouraging them to achieve their goals. Not everyone can pull it off. Chloe speaks of a friend who succeeded in doing just this.

CHLOE: *My friend Jack was very supportive of my weight loss, but he checked out how I was feeling. "How do you feel? Did you do this for other people, or are you doing it for yourself?" He thinks it's great, but he knows I'm a people pleaser, and he wanted to make sure I was doing it for the right reasons.*

This was Jack's way of communicating to Chloe that she was a wonderful person even if she did not change a thing. Although he was happy she was achieving her goal, he reminded her that she should do it because she wanted to and not for external approval. She is lovable, obese or not. Now that's a friend, and that's support! Not all of our interviewees were graced with that kind of companionship.

Some individuals reported being judged by friends for having taken the "easy way out," for giving in to what they perceived to be a quick surgical fix rather than accomplishing their weight loss through the traditional routes of dieting and exercise. The judgment was, essentially, that they were weak, that they lacked the character and willpower to lose weight the "right" way.

CANDACE: *My best friend of twenty-five years and I are not as close any-more. In fact, I have not talked to her in three weeks. She told my daugh-ter, "Your mom took the easy way out. She didn't try." And that really hurts me. It really hurt our relationship.*

This is not an uncommon judgment made about those who opt for obe-sity surgery. It is an extension of the societal prejudice about obesity being a sign of moral weakness. Even in the face of life-threatening conditions, some people still negatively judge those who opt for surgery. It is a testament to the true insidiousness of the prejudice. Even if we are dying, we really should continue trying to lose the weight using all those techniques that never worked for us before. Is the message, "Better to die knowing you were trying to do it through willpower than to live knowing that you surrendered to the surgery"? No one would put it quite that way, but that is essentially the message in this type of judgment. Besides, it is interesting to wonder whether the very people criticizing our interviewees for their choice would not take a magic pill themselves if it resulted in weight loss. Now *that* would be the easy way out. These harsh judgments also reveal a profound ignorance about the causes of extreme obesity and the factors that maintain it. They completely ignore all the research on genetics and metabolism and the complex emo-tional factors that collide to produce clinically severe obesity. Most impor-tant, this attitude grossly underestimates the amount of willpower needed to undergo the surgery and adhere to the strict lifelong diet that is an absolute requirement for success after obesity surgery.

TED: *I can sense in one particular friend a kind of dropping away. When I made the surgery decision, he had also decided to work on his weight but through dieting and exercise. He has worked very hard, and in a short pe-riod of time I have caught up to him, and I think this bothers him.*

If Ted's perception of his friend's feelings is correct, then his friend has not understood that Ted is also dieting and exercising. The only difference is that Ted made use of a tool that helped him be successful. And what is wrong with that?

Ted's alienation from his dieting friend touches on a theme that came up with a number of interviewees: the issue of relationships with friends who themselves are obese. After the surgery, some interviewees felt slightly uncomfortable with their obese friends because they feared their weight loss might make their friends feel bad or self-conscious. Prior to the weight loss, some of these folks described themselves and their obese friends as having a kind of sister- or brotherhood. They felt comfortable with each other, they could make fun of their weight good-heartedly, and they could complain together about the unpleasant aspects of being obese. A sort of camaraderie had developed around their shared problem. The fear then became that losing weight would in some way represent a betrayal of the group.

> CHLOE: *I have a friend who is very overweight (she's almost 400), and she came to visit recently. She's afraid I'm going to forget what it's like being overweight. I felt how uncomfortable she was being with me, and that made me sad because I'm like, "Don't think I'm different. I still love you. I don't care if you weigh 5,000 pounds. I'm still your friend."*

Weight loss in one person can also serve as a looking glass for obese friends. It can be experienced as increased pressure for them to also do something about their weight. If they are not ready to take steps, then it is quite possible that being with their weight-dropping friend will be experienced as unpleasant. Another wedge that is driven between the postsurgical patient and their obese friends is the fact that they start drifting toward different activities and sources of entertainment. Whereas many of their get-togethers might have been organized around food, now the person who's had the surgery cannot afford to be as invested in those activities. The situation is not unlike that of individuals who quit drinking or taking drugs. Hanging around friends who continue to do so can be problematic.

> GABRIELLE: *I guess I never realized that as a fat person I surrounded myself with fat friends, but I did. I ended up drifting apart from these friends, and I think it was entirely because of my weight loss because we just didn't do the same things we did before. A lot of times I also think it has to do with the attention I'll get compared to them.*

One disturbing, yet very common, report was the envy and resentment of some friends after the surgery. Many interviewees reported losing friends after surgery and attributed it primarily to resentment about their weight loss. It had upset the balance on which these relationships had apparently rested. At least, that was the perception of some of our interviewees.

CHLOE: *I've lost friends because of the weight loss. There's one friend who criticized me for having the surgery. In the last conversation we had, she asked why I had the surgery. I told her I wanted to be healthy. She said, "I don't think it's just to be healthy. I think you like the attention that you get now." I said, "No, it's because of my health. To be quite honest, I don't like the attention." She just didn't buy that. When we used to go out and do things, people would look at her because she was thinner. And now, if we were still friends, she would not be getting the attention. I think that's the problem.*

Sometimes the envy was framed as a joke, but some of our folks believed it to be serious, as they saw some of these relationships drift away.

DAPHNE: *Now that I'm losing weight, it's kind of like a joke—you know, "You bitch, you're looking pretty again"—but I do think my friends were more comfortable when I was not attractive to the men. I've noticed lately they don't call as often, and they don't e-mail as much. An obese person or an ugly person is not intimidating. So there are some friends who are secure and they accept me, and others who are insecure who are starting to reject me.*

Whether these friendships suffered because the weight loss was threatening or because our interviewees had in fact changed in other ways, it is clear that these friendships constituted a system in which obesity played a significant role. When the weight left, its role in the system was revealed.

ORIANNA: *I lost one good friend I used to also work with. This woman was wonderful to me before the surgery. She did all sorts of things for me at work and at home. Tremendously supportive when I was in hospital—even offered to take time off work when my husband, who had taken*

family leave to take care of me, had to return to work. But when our roles
changed, she couldn't take that. As I lost the weight, she no longer felt
needed. When the weight came off, I wanted to go out with her and actu-
ally do things. But she wasn't comfortable with that. She actually stopped
talking to me. I tried to reach her, saying, "Kim, what's wrong? Let's talk."
She'd reply, "No, no, nothing." And so I sent her a card, and I wrote, "I
must have said or done something to hurt you terribly. I don't know what
it is, so please can we talk?" She refused for a long time, and then finally
one day she agreed. She showed up with a long list of everything I had
done wrong, all my crimes. One of them was that I shouldn't twirl. And
I said, "What do you mean?" She said, "Well, everybody sees you losing
weight, and everyone sees you have new clothes, but on top of it you come
in and you twirl and you say, 'Look at me.' I don't need to see that. It both-
ers me." I tried to explain that after years of shopping out of Lane Bryant
or wearing clothes that fit but with no style or color that I loved show-
ing off my clothes. And I would twirl. She was jealous of my twirling . . .
strange situation. The friendship never made it past that. We tried, but it
just never worked again.

Now, we may think that Orianna's newfound ability to be active and feel good
about herself would make her a more satisfying friend. How could that be
anything but an improvement? However, for this friend it wasn't an improvement because her obesity played a very important role in this one friendship. It made Kim feel needed, important, and maybe even superior. Without
minimizing Kim's apparently impressive kindness toward Orianna prior to
and shortly after the surgery, the kindness was fulfilling a real need for Kim
also. A self-sufficient and attractive Orianna did not satisfy that deep need
in Kim. A happy, attractive Orianna left Kim without her important role in
her friend's life. Kim's objection to the "twirling" is also an incredibly vivid
illustration of how threatened she was by her friend's success. It is also a sad
story, because these two women had a great deal of feeling for each other at
one time. Yet when this particular system was reconfigured due to the weight
loss, it could not stand the strain. Kim was not able to find a place for herself

in the reconfiguration, despite Orianna's apparently heartfelt attempts to address the situation.

Some friends were quite unabashed about their declarations of distress regarding our interviewees' weight loss. It wasn't a question of interpretation—they came right out and told some of our interviewees that they didn't like the fact that they were thinner.

LAURA: *I had a neighbor who was a very, very close friend, and she no longer speaks to me. One day she brought me a pair of her jeans and said, "Here, try these on." And I was scared to try them on in case they were too tight and didn't fit, and I think she was banking on them not fitting me. But they did. I zipped them right up. She then told me that this bummed her out. And I didn't understand why. She said that she saw herself as considerably thinner than me and then realized she wasn't really. She was bummed out that her fat friend wore the same size as her.*

Gordon was pretty convinced he knew why this kind of thing happened.

GORDON: *I think some people like to hang around with people who are uglier than them, heavier than them, so they can feel superior. And when you start catching up to them in looks and size, they can become insecure.*

Now, in these cases, it would be easy to say, "Well, I guess these weren't real friends in the first place, so good riddance," but it's a lot more complicated than that. Had our interviewees not lost weight, they would have never experienced the limitations of these friendships. Whatever was motivating these presurgical friends, they still felt and behaved as good friends prior to the weight loss. They still held an important place in the lives of the people we interviewed. And thus, their loss was painful and disconcerting. It was much worse than losing a friend who had simply moved away. The loss was accompanied by the realization that the motives behind the friendship were less than golden in the first place. That constituted a double loss. First, and most obvious, they lost a future with friends they were anticipating sharing many more experiences with. But, second, they had also lost their past with these friends, because it made them reevaluate the true meaning of the relationship prior to the weight loss. This was difficult stuff.

The realization that some friendships had been dependent on the obesity was a total surprise for most of our interviewees. Others had some awareness that they might be being used by certain friends prior to the surgery, and they willfully chose to stop letting that happen.

> KARINA: *After I lost the weight I started analyzing some of my one-sided friendships. I felt I was the one who was always calling. I was the one who was always going out of my way. So, I just decided to be conscious of that and not make the next move. Let them call me. And you know what? The phone ain't ringing, and there was no other side to the friendships. So, some of my old friends have dropped by the wayside.*

> CHLOE: *I have another friend, Janie, who always wanted to hang out with the beautiful people. She used me because I was always at home. If she called, I was always available. If she wanted to talk, I would listen. And now, if she calls, I'm not available. I'm busy, I have other friends. So, I'm not able to meet her needs like she wants.*

Clearly, our interviewees hoped that if they started acting less accommodating, these friends would step up to the plate and prove that these relationships were in fact reciprocal. No one wants to be in a one-way relationship; no one wants to come to the realization that they were being used. However, when they were heavy, some of our interviewees let those relationships develop that way because it also served their purposes—they figured this was the best they could hope for. Now they wanted proof that their suspicions were wrong. But many did not get that proof, and it was painful to have their worst thoughts confirmed. In some cases, friends stopped calling with no explanation, whereas in others, friends experienced our interviewees' refusal to play by the old rules as hostile.

> PENELOPE: *I have lost some people because of this. I had a girlfriend who wrote me a very angry letter. "You're not the same nice, kind person you used to be. You've turned into a selfish bitch." I'm still that nice, kind*

person, but I'm not bending over the way I was before. I had to put my foot down and say, "I'm not going to give you what you want anymore because what you want diminishes me." I also had developed a relationship with a young woman, and she was looking for me to mother her in a lot of ways. And after the weight loss, I started seeing that I really wasn't doing anything more than giving in to all of her demands. It tugged on my heartstrings because I never had kids, and it would have been nice to have a nurturing relationship with a young woman. But I did things I never should have done, like give her a lot of money I was never going to get back, so I had to put my foot down.

So the system into which obesity once fit had been upset by the weight loss. The obesity had in some cases worked as a holding station for the caretaking needs of some friends and for the insecurity of others. It had also made our interviewees more likely to accept behavior they might not have accepted had they felt better about themselves. Their obesity and its associated consequences had made some of them feel lucky to have friends at all, so they did not quibble over things that bothered them, if and when they noticed them. After surgery, folks raised their friendship expectations, and some friends didn't measure up.

LAURA: *Truthfully, I think I've lost all my friends. I had them beating down my door. I was so popular. I couldn't keep up with the phone. I don't have anybody now. It makes me really sad, but I think that when you're fat, your expectations are lower. When you're fat, you let people take advantage of you, and when you lose the weight and stop letting this happen, you lose the friends.*

Some friendships survived our interviewees' gains in assertiveness and were even enriched by them. Some friends had truly not realized that they acted in unkind ways when the individual was obese. When confronted, they were able to own up to it, apologize, and try to act better in the future. Friendships that bore the strain of this type of evaluation and self-corrected were truly worth keeping and celebrating.

HELENA: *I have one really close friend who, at about the time I was hav-ing the surgery, made a comment about my little sports car. She said, "How come the fattest people always buy the smallest sports cars and try to fit into them?" At the time I replied, "Well, maybe because we like them as much as you size-8 petite women." But it really hurt me, and I kept it bot-tled up inside. We were at a restaurant one day after I had lost the weight, and I reminded her of this remark and said, "I went home and cried. You hurt my feelings, and you had no right because I am a person with feelings now and I had those same feelings when I weighed 300 pounds. To this day you owe me an apology for that, and I want it now." She looked at me and said, "Oh my God, I am sorry, and I promise I'll never hurt your feelings again." We are still great friends today!*

In useful contrast to these stories of friends being insensitive and even abusive at times with their obese friends, we also discovered cases in which our interviewees claimed they themselves were the abusive ones prior to the surgery. The unhappiness and low self-esteem that had accompanied the obesity had turned some people angry, hostile, and into "not very good friends." After the surgery, they felt better about themselves, and their behav-ior toward friends improved dramatically. For Ian, there was a lot of work ahead to try to make up for his meanness toward his friends when he was obese.

IAN: *After I lost the weight, I went back to try to repair some of the harm I had done with my friends when I was overweight. I was just mean—I wanted to blame someone else for my own misery. So I went back and talked to some close friends to try to make it up to them. It's helped a lot. My friends look at me and say they see a big change, and they tell me I'm a neat guy to deal with. I go out of my way to help them, just to be a better person, because I know how negative I was in the past.*

In these cases, friends responded with delight as our interviewees tried to make up for time lost and affection that had gone too long undemonstrated. The overwhelming result was a huge improvement in the quality of friendships, with increased openness, intimacy, and empathy. After all, when we hate ourselves and our life, it is difficult to be giving or to love anyone else. First, most of our resources are expended on trying to survive, and we have few resources left to distribute. Furthermore, we can't really believe anyone else would really like or love us, so we reject them before they have a chance to reject us. It is a defensive move that ends up in isolation and missed opportunities. After the surgery, some of our interviewees proclaimed they would never let that happen to them again.

> VANESSA: *I value my friends much more than I used to. It's not that they treat me differently. It's that I treat them differently. I think I was downright mean when I was heavier, especially to my thin friends because I resented their thinness. I resented the fact that my girlfriend could wear this little skimpy bathing suit while we were in Jamaica, and I'm wearing this stupid black thing with a skirt on it, which still made me look like a cow. And I could see that I wasn't nice to her. I had really good people in my life that I would find reasons not to be friends with. It was because I was ashamed of myself—I was embarrassed. Now I see myself opening up more and bringing these people back into my life and cherishing them.*

Shaking Up the Family

One of the major differences between family and friends is that we neither choose our family nor typically make decisions about which relatives we are going to keep. With few exceptions, usually related to childhood trauma, we are not likely to actively sever relations with members of our family. Even if at times it has crossed our minds, we generally work it out or simply try to live with our differences. For the most part, we stick with them through thick and thin. What binds families together can be made of all the right stuff (love, mutual concern, and respect) or of less desirable stuff (obligation or guilt). Regardless, the tie is strong, and it tends to weather conflict pretty resiliently. However, that does not mean that families are left unaffected by change in one member. Since our interviewees were adults who did not live with their families of origin, we did not expect the weight loss to cause a revolution, but we did wonder if they had noticed any significant reactions or changes.

Themes similar to those brought up in relation to friendships emerged here also, from support to lack of it, envy, and an increase in assertion and respect. One of the most positive responses was that, in becoming more healthy and independent, activity with the family had increased, and the sense of being a burden to them had decreased.

BRANDON: *I had some nieces and nephews who I was never able to play with, never able to babysit. Now I babysit with them, I cook for them. It certainly has affected them. I'm a lot more pleasant to be around because I am happier, so it has affected my family a lot. Now they can depend on me. They don't have to assist me like they used to. Before, I would have to have somebody from my family run all my errands or go to the bank or go grocery shopping for me. It's given them freedom because they don't have to worry about me. It has brought me closer to them because I no longer feel like a burden.*

Another common report was that the individual's standing within the family had changed. They had gained respect through their weight loss. In some individuals whose families had previously engaged in open insults, the change was dramatic.

CHLOE: *My father would always belittle me before, but he does not do that anymore. He used to call me stupid, even though I am the most educated person in my family, but his attitude is different now. My brother and sister are also more respectful now. My brother used to say "Fat slob," and I don't hear that anymore. I think they were a little envious of me, because I was a good student and my parents saved their money for me to go to college instead of them. But I don't hear comments like that from them anymore.*

Families of origin are perhaps the most difficult systems to change. In one way, this makes them the most resilient and least likely to break down when change in one member occurs. However, that is in part because denial of change is strongest in family systems. The roles that develop in families of origin are long-standing—they developed a long time ago, and since most of us leave home relatively early on, the family is not exposed on a daily basis to the changes we have undergone. Occasional visits back home do not seem to provide sufficient proof that a reconfiguration of roles may be called for. Families often complain of us putting on airs or acting strangely because they still expect the "old" person—the person who left. They have not lived through or witnessed the changes. The original role thus tends to persist doggedly and sometimes against all manner of disconfirming information. That is one of the reasons that people often feel they are regressing when they go home or that no one knows who they really are.

In order to effect the change they needed from their families of origin, some of our interviewees simply started acting more assertively. This change alone made them reconfigure old patterns of behavior within the family.

LAWRENCE: *My position in the family has definitely changed. I don't know what it is, can't put my finger on it, but it's changed. I don't put up with as much from them. My sisters would henpeck me to death. And I think I stand up for myself now.*

Abby recounted one showdown with her mother-in-law that would have been inconceivable to her prior to the weight loss.

ABBY: *My mother-in-law is living with us, and I decided to show her my list of demands or rules while she is living with us. I was scared to death, but losing the weight has given me the courage to do what needs to be done. It was hard, but I gave her the list of the things that I need. I sat there for a moment and waited to see if she had any questions. I got up and walked out. I didn't try to justify or give reasons why. "This is what I expect." I would have never had the courage when I was heavy.*

But there was still resistance. There is always resistance to change in systems, even when the change is positive. In families, this resistance manifested itself in a number of ways reminiscent of what had happened in friendships, although with much less dramatic outcomes. In the cases of families with more than one obese member, the individual's surgery and weight loss were experienced with some discomfort by those who either needed to take some action or needed the individual to remain heavy as a form of positive contrast to themselves.

> GABRIELLE: *It's affected my relationship with my mom. She's overweight also but not as much as I was. All I ever heard was, "Don't you feel it's time to take the weight off?" and now it's, "Don't you think you're just a little too thin?"*

Here was Gabrielle finally accomplishing what her mother had always said she wanted her to accomplish, but instead of reinforcement, she gained concern about maybe being too thin. We can imagine the frustration of this. It is one of those situations in which many people feel trapped with their parents—that somehow we can never make them happy. On the other hand, the weight loss after gastric bypass surgery is so rapid and dramatic that it is entirely possible that Gabrielle's mother was starting to become genuinely concerned. That is not, however, how Gabrielle experienced it.

The weight loss also served to highlight the weight problems of other members of the family. Whereas our interviewees felt a strong need to talk about their accomplishment, certain family members did not want to partake of these discussions because it made them feel bad about themselves.

> DAPHNE: *Most of my family has been supportive, but my mother is in denial. She would rather not discuss my weight loss. She does not realize she has a weight problem too. She doesn't share in my happiness, and that hurts because when you feel you were near death and lost so much and then get a second chance at life, you can't help but want to brag.*

Some family members even pulled out the now-familiar refrain about surgery being "the easy way out" as a way of defending against their own lack of action. Sisters seemed to figure prominently in these types of reactions. Some of the ones who were themselves overweight withdrew from our interviewees, whereas others who were very invested in being the thinner sister felt their identity and role within the family threatened by the weight loss.

> MAGGIE: *My sister withdrew from me when I started losing weight. She was always the slender one in the family, and as I lost weight she started to gain some. She started to pull back. Sometimes you have to let people go.*

The outcome in Maggie's case was particularly upsetting, as she ended up losing touch with her sister altogether. Now, it is quite probable that Maggie and her sister had a whole set of problems that had nothing to do with the weight loss, but the weight loss seems to have driven the final wedge into their relationship. Reactions such as these were very surprising to our interviewees. Not one of them had predicted that the reactions from their families would be anything but gleeful. Other sisters navigated this crisis to a more successful resolution.

> ORIANNA: *My sister also had weight problems. She had lost and regained her weight several times. Right now she's at her highest weight ever. Well, she couldn't look at me after my surgery. She lives only blocks away, but I hardly saw her when I started losing weight. I could see it was envy. Her mouth would say she was proud of me, that she was happy for me, but I could see the looks. I really felt bad for her, and I didn't know how to deal with it. It probably took us about a year to come to terms with it.*

> VANESSA: *My sister is supportive but also a little envious. She keeps on telling me I've lost enough, but I think what she's really saying is, "Don't lose 15 pounds more because then you'll weigh less than me."*

It is not surprising that sibling relationships were so affected by the change in our interviewees, considering that these are usually the closest family relationships. If anyone was going to feel the role change, it would be a sister.

In other cases, the surgery and weight loss motivated overweight family members to also finally do something about their own weight problems. This was experienced very positively. Surgery had helped them accomplish what their families had always wanted them to do, but, better yet, it had also turned them into role models.

> FRANCES: *My decision to have the surgery was a wake-up call to my mom, who was also overweight. She was amazed at what I achieved and real supportive, and it made her decide she also needed to do something with her life. So, it's been kind of cool.*

And so, to summarize, very few relationships went unchanged when the weight started to drop. Marriages deteriorated or thrived, mostly depending on the quality of the relationship prior to surgery. Our impression was that marriages that were strong to begin with became better, whereas those built on an unsteady foundation were not able to bear the quake of dramatic weight loss. The effect on sexual relationships was interesting in that pretty much everyone agreed that sex was easier, though a surprising number of the women in our group spoke of a loss of desire. Children were delighted, as they got their parents back or maybe even got them fully for the first time. Friendships were perhaps the most reactive to the weight loss, with major shake-ups in most people's friendship networks. And finally, families reacted in a variety of ways, with most of them settling in to the new reality relatively successfully over time.

CHAPTER 4 | **Deconstructing the Self**

Who Was I and Who Am I Becoming?

What did I become because of the obesity?
And now what can I become?
—PENELOPE

You get wheeled into the operating room, and the surgeon's scalpel dramatically alters your gastrointestinal system so that when you exit, it is physically impossible to eat anywhere near the amounts you ate before. You simply get violently ill if you try. The result is rapid weight loss. Great! Fabulous! The ultimate fantasy! At least for a while. But as Mona so aptly put it, "When the doc does this surgery, he doesn't do a lobotomy—he changes your body, not your brain." Obesity surgery is most definitely not brain surgery. Your personhood remains untouched by that scalpel, at least initially. The way you define yourself, your self-concept, your hopes, your insecurities, your strengths, your weaknesses, the mental and emotional effects of having been obese for a lifetime—none of those things are excised or stapled or reduced during those few hours in the operating room.

> MONA: *Ninety percent of the fat is between your ears. It's in your brain.*
> *I think that's what I have to work on: changing the fat mentality. I mean,*
> *I'm a size 10 and I still think I'm fat, and that's insane.*

As you lose the weight, your mind has to process the experience of your new body. Readjusting to a new body means readjusting to a different way of living and to a multitude of changes in the way the world reacts to you. For this reason, obesity surgery is often followed by much self-reflection and a reevaluation of both past and future in regards to self-concept. This surgery is not like getting a polyp excised or a mole removed. Those surgeries don't make us wonder what we became, who we really are, and who we want to be. Obesity surgery radically changes us on a dimension that others are both highly conscious of and judgmental about—the way we look. It seems inevitable that that change would shine a spotlight on questions of self. Beauty may be only skin deep, but tell that to our interviewees. They'll tell you that the effects of obesity and then weight loss went far deeper than that. The effects went down to their very cores—to the essence of their self-definitions.

In the past couple of chapters, we focused on the dramatically different way that both strangers and intimates related to our interviewees. There seems little doubt that many relationships experienced significant adjustments. However, the most significant psychological impact of the surgery was on the individual's construction of self—their self-concept. The word *construction* here is important because part of what the surgery brings to light is that our self-concept is something we, in part, build. It is not exclusively an essential aspect of who we "are"; self is also a lifelong work in progress shaped by what happens to us and how we interpret it.

Research shows that certain basic aspects of our personalities may be biologically determined.[1] Characteristics such as shyness or extraversion or emotional reactivity are witnessed in infants very early on, and these characteristics seem to be personality traits that are fairly constant over time. Some characteristics, such as reactivity, which is essentially high emotional sensitivity, can be evidenced in babies only days old. Research that follows people over many years (longitudinal) indicates that these characteristics persist and are, to some extent, surprisingly unaffected by parenting and other environmental influences. So it seems pretty clear that we may be born with a tendency toward some of the broadly drawn lines of our personalities. Shy children are more likely to grow up to be socially anxious adults than children who are not shy. However, the specifics of a person's life also affect biology. Whether a child is born with a predisposition to shyness or to extraversion, both of these traits are going to be impacted to some extent by environmental influences. So an emotionally reactive child reared in a secure, calm, and loving environment is going to have this emotional reactivity attenuated in adulthood. This kind of environment will calm that person down. On the other hand, if the child is reared in a chaotic, emotionally volatile environment, it is likely that his or her predisposition will be further magnified.

Clinically severe obesity is both a biological and an environmental phenomenon. It is biological because (1) there is a genetic predisposition to it,[2] and (2) extreme obesity significantly alters physiological functions. It is also an environmental phenomenon because (1) it is influenced dramatically by environmental circumstances,[3] and (2) it has a tremendous impact on the way that the world reacts to us. In our society, obesity creates a pretty significant environmental influence. It may or may not rise to the level of abuse or trauma or neglect, but it is rarely negligible. An obese child is likely to be ostracized and ridiculed, no matter his or her basic personality. Even if the child was born with a tendency toward being extraverted and gregarious, getting negative feedback from the world is likely to affect how that child sees him- or herself, as well as how he or she sees others. Thus, early on in life, self-concept starts to be constructed on top of whatever the genetic tendency toward a personality style might have been. An inherent predisposition to extraversion may be curtailed by the social rejection created by the obesity. Conversely, a predisposition toward shyness may be magnified by these same negative influences in the obese child or adult.

At different points in their journey out of obesity, our interviewees came to appreciate how certain parts of their self-concept had been constructed over a lifetime. Some characteristics changed, and others stubbornly persisted, even after their lives had changed so dramatically. As the weight dropped, some individuals reported that their view of "who they were" started to feel a little shaky. They experienced something akin to an identity crisis. Others had trouble shaking old traits and assumptions that they had once attributed to the obesity. Now that they were significantly smaller, they discovered that those traits were not going away. Paradoxically, sometimes it's easier to build than it is to tear down. For some of our interviewees, a construction of self that had been many years in the making was not going to dissolve as easily as the sutures from the surgery. For others, the change in self-perception was so swift that it left them confused and wondering who the heck they were. In both cases, the weight loss seemed to lead back to questions about self. The archetypal "Who am I?" question was a very serious one indeed for many of our interviewees.

How Could I Have Let Myself Get to This?

The first wave of self-reflection was to wonder how they had let themselves get as obese as they had been presurgery. They reflected on what that said about them. Presurgery, many of them had gotten to the stage at which they considered their weight an inevitability—something completely outside of their control. Being heavy was just the way it was. Nothing to be done. The surgery and the strict dietary regimen they then found themselves adhering to had shattered that illusion of inevitability. Think about it: After the surgery, they had to be on a very intense dietary regimen that is experienced as quite difficult even with a new, restricted stomach. If they could maintain that diet now, why had they not successfully maintained a diet before? In many cases, the doctor would refuse to operate until the patient had proven that he or she could lose a certain amount of weight in the six months prior to the surgery. And by "proven," we mean that the doctor would send the patient home and say that he would not schedule the operation until the patient came back 50 or more pounds lighter. This was a confusing turn of events for Frances and a number of other folks we interviewed. After all, why would they be opting for the operation if they could diet successfully?

> FRANCES: *The doctor told me I would have to lose 50 pounds before he would touch me, and he just cut me loose and told me to come back when I had done that. I thought he was going to fix me and everything would be okay. Now I was faced with the idea that I had to fix me first before he would have me on that operating table. I thought, "Well, if I could do that, I would have done it in the past, so what the hell am I going to do?"*

Dr. Fisher's rationale for requesting weight loss prior to the surgery was twofold. First, he knew that the heavier the patient, the greater the risk of surgical complications. If he could get some of the most severely obese patients to lose some of the weight presurgically, their chances for better immediate surgical outcomes rose significantly.[4] Second, he also knew that, postsurgically, they would have to adhere to a difficult diet, and he wanted to test their commitment and build their self-efficacy for dieting. The reactions to this request for presurgical weight loss were often very emotional. Prospective patients often cried in desperation and became quite angry with the surgeon. But he stuck to his guns because he knew it was in their best interest.

Despite her initial reaction, Frances did indeed lose weight before the surgery. She actually lost 10 more pounds than the doctor had requested. And that was a little confusing. She wondered if she shouldn't just stay on the diet, but she was afraid of backsliding and decided to opt for the surgery. However, having lost those 60 pounds preoperatively left her with questions about why she had never been successful before. How could she have let herself slide into severe obesity when she had just proven that she could in fact control it? On the other hand, the presurgical weight loss had had the very important effect of giving her strength for the postsurgical efforts. And that's what Dr. Fisher had intended.

FRANCES: *Losing those 60 pounds has served me so well over the eighteen months since the surgery. Just knowing that I could do it. That I could stay on a diet.*

Liposuction, a surgical procedure that individuals undergo to remove excess fat, would not have had the effect of making people wonder about their control, because liposuction does not require any effort on the part of the patient. After recovering from surgery, there are no real directives about how to live or eat. Gastric bypass surgery removes no fat. It reduces the size of the stomach and rearranges your intestines and then commits you to a diet you would have never believed you could stick to. Initially, the surgery makes it easier to diet because the stomach cannot handle as much. But remember the brain! We still *want* that chocolate sundae; we'd still kill for that bag of chips! So after obesity surgery, we are on a very strict diet that, no matter how small our new stomach pouch, will always be a challenge to stay on. It still requires an enormous amount of planning, commitment, and willpower. When our interviewees found that they could indeed stand down this willpower challenge after the surgery, it brought them face-to-face with the choices they had made over a lifetime. They wondered why they had not had the will to do something about it earlier—be it surgery or the dietary regimen they now found themselves on anyway.

> BRANDON: *What I find amazing and have no answer for is why did I and why do other people let themselves get to this point? It wasn't really a process I could see evolving. I woke up one day, and there it was. But obviously it didn't happen that way. It took several years to get to the weight I was. And I never realized that it was happening until all of a sudden there it was. Maybe I was ignoring it. I don't know. But I was disappointed that I let it get that far—to the point of no control.*

It is interesting that Brandon "didn't see it coming." Did he really not see it happening, or did he see it but think little of it because it happened so incrementally? One pound today, another tomorrow. It isn't that hard to imagine how one would pay little attention on a daily basis yet find oneself unrecognizable a few years hence. The limitations build up slowly, one on top of the other over many years. We start getting used to them. We feel normal and, without realizing it, go from preferring not to walk somewhere to not being able to tie our shoes. We even stop tracking the multitude of things we can no longer do. Many of our interviewees expressed that they were not aware of how many limitations they were living with until the weight loss started doing away with them.

> RONALD: *Just realizing where I've been, what I gave up, what I was doing to myself! Now I see the freedom available to me, and the difference is night and day.*

Maybe it wasn't that they didn't notice, but that they did not want to acknowledge it. Maybe they were seeing it happen out of the corner of their eyes but decided not to pay attention because that would involve trying to tackle a problem they felt helpless to overcome. It was an effort in which they were not ready to invest. This seems probable considering their level of disappointment with themselves. Yet who among us can claim not to have acted similarly when what we needed to do was so difficult? That's what rationalization is all about.

> FRANCES: *When I applied to architecture school, it was the first time I felt forced to confront the role that being morbidly obese was really playing in my life. I don't know if before I was just oblivious. I was so oblivious that in my prior job as a dental hygienist I convinced myself that the work was not very intellectually challenging when in fact it was the physical demands of the work that I could not bear because of my weight.*

We concoct a really good reason to do something we should not be doing rather than do the right thing, plain and simple. That's because the right thing is usually neither plain nor simple. This feeling of shame for having let things get so bad was common among our interviewees. Talia remembers saying to her husband, "Shame on me for letting me and letting you get away with the things that I did for so many years!"

It seems a testament to the human desire for self-knowledge and understanding that once out of the fire, we still have a need to know what got us there in the first place. It would be easy enough to say, "Phew, got out of that bind!" and leave it at that. Yet we often do not. We feel a need to know what drove us there. We feel a need to understand what factors contributed to or resulted in us being in such a terrible situation. Is it because we don't want to repeat the mistake, or is it because, even when it serves no instrumental purpose, we simply want to better know ourselves? Maybe a little of both. Either way, our interviewees thought long and hard about their responsibility in letting themselves get extremely obese. None of them fell back on genetic explanations, reasonable though that would have been in some cases. The need to understand their role in the development of their obesity, as well as their lack of agency prior to the surgery, was pretty much ubiquitous. No one said to themselves, "Oh, well, who cares how I got that way? I'm not like that anymore."

> KARINA: *I think back now to my typical day before the surgery versus what it is today, and I just shake my head. I can't believe I ever let myself live that way.*

Maybe one of the answers to how they were able to let themselves get that obese lies in the fact that they had no idea how different life could be. One can guess that an effective self-defense would be to imagine that things would not be that different without the weight. No big deal! Obese, not obese. How different can that be? Well, when they were losing the weight and experiencing dramatic change in just about every aspect of their lives, they learned the answer—life could be very different indeed! Many of the changes were small, but they added up. Being able to tie their shoes, to wash themselves easily, to sit on the floor, to play with their kids, and so on.

RONALD: *The realization of what the obesity took away, what I let happen over the years, dawned on me about six months after the surgery. I had not really realized what I had done to myself.*

The contrast between pre- and postsurgical life was not just something to rejoice in but, more important, something to understand. Losing weight was simply not enough. People needed to understand what had gotten them in that state in the first place and what had prevented them from changing their circumstances. The need to know seemed unstoppable.

MAGGIE: *When the surgery started to change my whole life, I went back and took stock regarding why I was the way I was. You need to go back and look at everything in your life, what got you to that point, why you had the surgery, and what it's doing to you.*

Some people felt the need to see a therapist to work it all out. This was their new project. The problem with their bodies had been addressed by the surgery, the problems that may have contributed to their obesity called for a different type of intervention.

ERICA: *I've started seeing a therapist because I need to understand the issues that led me to be obese.*

LAWRENCE: *I go to counseling to deal with the self-esteem issues and to get coping skills.*

A number of our interviewees who pondered the reasons they had let themselves get to the point of clinically severe obesity reached the conclusion that the obesity had simply been the defensive strategy of defeatism. They had convinced themselves that nothing could be improved—that nothing could ever get better.

TALIA: *I should have done this a long time ago, but, unfortunately, I had already planned that my life was going to be hell.*

It may seem strange that we can find comfort in defeatism, as it seems so grim an idea. However, giving up does have its benefits. Primarily, it lets us off the hook from working and struggling to improve our situation. Miserable though our circumstances may be, we can come to think that trying to improve them could be even worse. It would surely mean hard work, and it might result in failure. Most often this is not even a conscious process. We don't have a sense of having made a decision to give up; we just do. The familiar does have its comforts. If we don't try to improve things, then we won't experience failure—other than, of course, the even bigger failure of not aiming higher. Yet somehow, the failure of not trying can come to be perceived as potentially less painful than that of trying and maybe not making it.

Another paradoxical reaction to negative circumstances is that we can actually become somewhat attached to the misery. Attached to misery? How can that be? Well, if we have organized our entire life and identity around one set of circumstances, we may not be able to envision life any other way. We may also be afraid that we wouldn't know "how to be" any other way. Obesity can shield us from romantic experiences, occupational challenges, or even finding out who we really are, apart from the fat. We may be missing out on a lot, but it may feel safer. Living less usually means risking less. Some folks can get to the point of thinking that living half a life is more comfortable than taking their chances on a full one.

Who Might I Have Become?

Along with a substantial amount of the self-reflection about the past came a feeling of regret for time and opportunities lost. For some folks, this was a very sad experience. They started to feel very sorry for the people they were before the surgery.

TALIA: *I didn't think I was that fat when I looked at myself before, but now that I've lost 92 pounds and I look at old pictures, it hurts me and makes me cry because I never saw it.*

Why was Talia crying then? Who was she crying for? It seems that Talia was crying because when she looked at old photographs, she saw herself as other people had. She felt very sad for the person she was. Talia was crying for the person who was so tragically oblivious to the fact that she was extremely obese, who was blind to the fact that people were not seeing her as she saw herself. It is interesting that we can cry for the people we were. In the case of our interviewees, it illustrates the splitting of the self into the postsurgical person and the presurgical one. One can now weep for the previous self the way one would for a loved friend we could not help in a sad situation. It is a type of delayed reaction to the pain they were actually experiencing at the time. Maybe it is only with the weight loss that it feels safe to truly feel the pain of their obesity circumstances. Giving in to the pain when they were stuck in the obesity might have been paralyzing. With the weight loss came the luxury of crying over something you had now changed and mastered. But it remained heartbreaking and could elicit tears in many of the people we interviewed years after the surgery.

For some individuals, the postsurgical period also brought about an enormous sense of loss and waste. They now fully appreciated all the years they had let pass without attempting to fulfill dreams and aspirations simply because the weight was in the way. With that realization came regret.

BRANDON: *I wish I would have done it earlier because there are a lot of years that have been wasted as a result of being heavy and not being able to do a lot of things.*

An interesting corollary of this historical revisionism—this looking at the past in a different way—is to wonder what your life would have been like, if you had either never been overweight or had lost the weight a long time ago. Imagining a different past was a common thought process shortly after the surgery.

ABBY: *When I was young, my doctor recommended that I lose 40 pounds before going on the student-exchange program. So I ended up not going on the program. I went to college out of state instead and got married there, but I always wonder how my life could have been totally different if I had been just a little thinner.*

Would Abby have married someone else? Might she not have married at all? Might her career have been completely different? We all wonder the extent to which our lives would have been different had we gone to a different school or taken a different vacation, for example. There is a film starring Gwyneth Paltrow called *Sliding Doors* that examines this issue directly. The film basically explores what her character's life would have been had a certain subway door closed, compared to what it would have been had that very door stayed open a few seconds longer and she had been able to board the subway car. The question at the heart of this film is how differently might our lives have turned out had we done one little thing differently or, even more pointedly, had some random event intervened—a random event such as a subway door closing as you were about to get on and perhaps meet your future husband. There seems little question that at least some aspects of our lives are determined by little accidents or random events. Wondering about the effects of these can be a whimsical, daydreaming kind of question. But to our interviewees, that question was very real. Their obesity had led them to choices that were likely to have been very different from those available to them had they not been obese. However, unlike in the case of the sliding subway door, our interviewees did not think their obesity had been determined by chance. Judging by their high levels of self-blame, most felt a great deal of responsibility for their weight and how it had determined their life course.

Although a number fantasized about lives of greater achievement had they not been obese, some wondered quite the opposite. We do not often think about conditions of adversity leading to achievement, particularly when we are in the thick of the adversity. But, in retrospect, some folks started to seriously consider the possibility that the weight had actually made them excel in some areas. Others wondered if the obesity itself had kept them on some moral, straight-and-narrow path. Had they felt more physically attractive, might they have taken an easier, less achievement-oriented path?

FRANCES: *I wonder if I would have been thin and cute throughout high school and adolescence, would I have become a stripper or something? What would I have done? Would I just have gotten married straight out of high school and not gone to college? Would I have fought so hard to achieve? I don't think so. Because now that I've lost the weight I don't feel as compulsive. I don't feel I have to be the straight-A student. I'm okay with a B now because I feel okay about myself in general. Achievement is not that personal anymore.*

It is unlikely that Frances's proverbial fork in the road presented two such extreme directions as either that of obese overachiever or that of thin stripper. On the other hand, it is perfectly believable that the handicap of weight led her to compensate for this "weakness" by developing other strengths. Many people who perceive themselves as deficient in one area report overachieving in another. It is also hard to dismiss Frances's own observation that once she lost the weight, she did not care as much about excelling in school. Although it is unlikely that a thin Frances would have become a stripper, it is quite probable that the obesity provided an extra dose of motivation to succeed professionally. It is, however, interesting that she pits professional success against stripping. She does not contrast professional success with professional failure, but rather with a blatantly sexual way of earning a living. This may just have been a manner of speaking, but she was not the only one to wonder if the only thing standing between her and a more promiscuous or sexually focused lifestyle was the obesity.

PENELOPE: *Who can you be now? Do you go back? There's really no going back. But what would you have been? Less of a good girl, perhaps?*

CANDACE: *What if I go cheat on my husband? I don't know what I'm capable of.*

It is possible that these women were a little heady with the sexual attention they were receiving after a lifetime of being treated as completely asexual, if not antisexual. It was a powerful experience to be considered sexy when most of their past experiences with men had ranged anywhere from neglect to mocking. The power of this newfound attention led a few of our women to wonder what they would have done with the positive attention had they experienced it early on. Their concerns about the possibility of having become promiscuous or having led a life driven primarily by sexual concerns are probably a gross miscalculation. Most nonobese women learn to live with the sexual attention, and they judge it for what it is from adolescence into adulthood. It does not feel as precious as it might to a woman who has never had that kind of attention—it is part of what they grew up with. On occasion, they probably find it annoying, or even at times threatening. Most women do not end up becoming strippers, and those who do would probably laugh at the implication that they strip for a living because of the irresistible lure of being found sexually attractive. Most women do not become sexually promiscuous, and those who do probably have a variety of reasons for this behavior, only one of which might be the pleasure of being desired.

This concern about what their sexual behavior would have been without the weight is a perfect example of how obesity impacts men and women differently. No man we interviewed expressed concerns about having ended up a "bad boy" had he not been very obese. Clearly, this illustrates the double standard that our society still has about sexual behavior in men and women. The women worried about becoming too sexual, but the men did not. The men may have wondered if they would have gotten more dates without the weight, but not one of them wondered whether the weight was the one thing that had kept them from a life of unbridled and negatively judged sexual activity. They did, however, also express a sense of not being sure where the weight loss would lead in terms of who they would become, more generally speaking.

GORDON: *Who knows where I might end up? There are other problems out there, you know?*

For our recently operated-on interviewees, there was definitely a palpable sense of uncertainty about the future and who they would become. At times, all this wondering about future outcomes sounded uncannily like the musings of children who are trying to figure out "what they want to be when they grow up." And that is not because our interviewees were immature. These were generally accomplished and thoughtful individuals who had been through a lot. However, they were new to a life in which they were not severely obese. In that sense, they were innocent. They did not know what that life might hold in store for them. They had been reborn, and they simply wondered what lay ahead.

Is It Them or Is It Me?

As patients experienced changes in relationships with their families, coworkers, and strangers, they often wondered who in fact was changing—them or the people around them. It was not at all clear, and the question nagged at them. Getting the answer right seemed to be of great importance, as they brought it up repeatedly in very similar ways.

> CHLOE: *I am the same person. I am just as educated. I am just as friendly. I haven't changed my values. They are the same. So I just really think it's them changing more than me. But then I recognize that I do feel better about myself, and I probably do project that.*

Here it sounds as if Chloe wants to think that she has not changed—that the only difference is her weight. She once weighed 300 pounds, and now she weighs 165. Period. Yet she has this gnawing feeling that because of the weight loss, she has in fact changed internally. She feels better about herself and intuitively imagines that this gain in self-esteem is translating into a more positive pattern of behavior that the world is responding to. Many of our interviewees reported that people often commented on how different they seemed after the weight loss, and not just physically.

On the other hand, not everyone noticed a difference in the reactions and treatment of others. Folks who did not experience a noticeable change wondered if it was the lingering effect of having once been obese that kept things the same. They wondered if others continued to see them as obese long after they had lost the weight. Did the fat follow them around like a halo, like the slight trace of a drawing that has been erased but still shows on the paper?

ERICA: *I still have the same issues at work that I had before the surgery. I still don't have the promotion I wanted, and I wonder if it's because they still see me as a fat person who they want to keep in the back office or if it's my personality they don't like.*

It might have been a little premature only nine months after the surgery for Erica to expect big changes, but then again other folks spoke of these changes happening even sooner. Erica was clearly struggling with the "Is it me or is it them?" question that is really at the heart of all honest reflections on interpersonal interactions. It is definitely easier to blame interpersonal difficulties on "them." However, it is neither the most sincere nor the most useful thing to do. Every interaction requires the participation of at least two parties, and thus every interaction is characterized and affected by the actions and feelings of both parties.

KARINA: *Not having that weight enables me to think a different way, which enables people to see me in a different way.*

People are generally nice to people who are nice to them and vice versa. Some folks out there are unkind to severely obese people, regardless of whether the obese person is nice or not. We know that. However, it is probably a pretty good bet to assume that obese people who are nice to others are probably treated better on average than those who either engage in social avoidance or act in antisocial ways. That was certainly the story we heard from our interviewees.

QUINCY: *Before it didn't matter if you liked me. Now that I'm a littler person, I want you to like me.*

When Quincy started caring about being liked, he started acting more positively toward others, which made others behave better with him.

Asking the "Is it me or is it them?" question is a tough but sophisticated thing to do. It is also the most successful route to self- and relationship improvement. Usually, the truest response to that question is, "It's both." That was the conclusion of a number of the individuals we spoke to.

> CHLOE: *People's perceptions of me have changed, but also my perceptions of them have changed. I feel they are more accepting of me, respect me more, value my opinion. So, I don't know if I've changed, which allowed them to change, or it all has to do with their perception of overweight people. I want to believe it's because I changed, and that that is the reason they changed their opinion of me.*

Chloe was here concluding that the change had been mutual, yet unlike in her immediately previous statement, she expressed a desire for the change to have been hers primarily. She "wanted to believe" that. But why might Chloe have been so invested in the idea that she was the one who had changed instead of them? Well, if their opinion of her was not contingent on how she was acting and feeling, then it meant that it was contingent on the weight alone. Understandably, Chloe did not want to believe that the world could be that superficial and that unkind. It was easier for her to take some responsibility. The discrepancy between Chloe's conclusion and what she wished were true is important because it illustrates nicely that we are often invested in certain explanations, even when we are honestly trying to figure something out. Some explanations are simply easier to live with than others.

Brandon also struggled with the hurtful possibility that the reaction from others was all weight-based. He finally concluded that it couldn't be—that he had indeed changed dramatically.

> BRANDON: *How can all the discrimination just disappear with the weight loss? I mean, I'm the same person that I've always been. I mean, some things have obviously changed physically and mentally. But then again, I guess I'm not the same person because I have totally redone the person. My attitudes are different, my feelings are different, my looks are different. So if I were to pick up and move somewhere else, I'd be a whole different person no one had ever known before.*

'lhe bottom line here is that the answer to the question, "Is it me or is it them?" carries with it some important implications about the self and about the world. If it's me, then it means that something as seemingly superficial as a few or many pounds of flesh has the power to determine the kind of person I am. Yikes! That will shatter a lot of the illusions you may have about what determines your heart and soul. On the other hand, if it's them, then it means that you live in a world that constructs an impression of you almost entirely based on your appearance—you are how you look. That's also kind of difficult to swallow!

In any case, the personal change seemed to come as a surprise for many of the folks we spoke to. For the most part, it was experienced as positive but challenging. It was a lot of change in a short period of time, and the sheer unpredictability of it rocked a lot of lives. They had not expected to experience such dramatic internal upheaval, and the nature of the changes that came about was nothing short of shocking.

MAGGIE: *You go into the surgery thinking that once you lose the weight things will get better. The bad will disappear. You'll be able to handle life differently, and everyone will accept you, and things will be glorious. And what you don't realize at the time is that it changes some of the people around you, but it changes you more greatly than anyone else. It changes how you feel and how you react to things.*

In contrast, a couple of interviewees were convinced that they were acting no differently after the surgery. They had little trouble chalking up all the new positive attention to the fact that people were finally taking notice of them simply because the weight had come off. Irma felt no conflict in this regard whatsoever. Being better treated was all that mattered. She did not care why or how it had happened. She was convinced it was others who had changed and was not the least bit interested in their explanations for that change.

IRMA: *I personally don't feel that I have changed. I'm as outspoken as ever. I'm just taking advantage of the fact that they are listening to me now, because they* think *I have changed.*

Perhaps the most intriguing aspect of the "Is it me or is it them?" question is that it highlights how difficult it is to tease apart our self-concept from the concept others have of us. We want to believe that we are self-defining, self-determining individuals, but the truth is that we are, at least in part, a reflection of what others see. From the moment of birth, when our mom first holds us in her arms, until our dying moments, we are dependent on social confirmation of our value. People vary in the extent to which they are affected or defined by the reactions of others, but no one comes close to completely escaping the social construction of who they are. Our gastric bypass patients had a particularly sharp insight into this because they were in the unusual situation of seeing everything around them change as a function of one stomach operation. They had the benefit of the "before and after" perspective that most other people don't get to witness. This perspective broke down a lot of illusions about the extent to which self-concept is an individualistic enterprise.

Will My Brain Ever Catch Up?

Usually, the process of losing weight by conventional methods is painfully long, slow, and plodding. We diet, we deprive ourselves, and the next morning we have either lost nothing or what feels like too small an amount for the effort we've made. It often simply feels as if it's not working and definitely not working fast enough. It can be terribly disheartening. So much effort for what feels like so small an improvement from day to day! The reinforcement of weight loss for all of our self-deprivation seems excruciatingly small and slow in coming. In the case of obesity surgery, though, the weight loss happens very quickly. The people we interviewed shortly after the surgery had already lost enormous amounts of weight. In six months, Talia had lost 92 pounds. In eight months, Brandon had lost 90, whereas Jessica and Karina had lost more than 200 pounds each. In nine months, Erica had lost 145. Within months of the surgery, our interviewees were shedding the weight equivalent of a whole other person. Nothing slow and plodding about that! However, psychologically adapting to the weight loss was another matter.

That, ironically, lagged way behind the weight loss. The weight came off their bodies at a shockingly quick pace, but many still felt they had the mind of a fat person.

Think about it: Suppose you have been extremely obese for all or a good part of your life. It is *who* you have been for a long time. It has likely had an impact on your self-definition, how you view and judge yourself, how you explain some or many of the things that have happened to you. And even if you are not someone who incorporated the weight into their self-definition, you have probably thought that others defined you as such, at least sometimes. You have spent a lifetime bracing yourself for the reactions of strangers. You knew when you walked into a public area that some would stare and others would purposely look away. You have maybe turned a deaf ear to the less-than-kind things said about you either to your face or behind your back just loud enough for you to hear. You have wondered how people close to you *really* feel about your weight, even as they tell you you're beautiful to them. Are they just being kind? Any one or all of these things are likely to add up to a schema about self and others largely defined by your weight. By schema, we mean a whole collection of thoughts and attitudes and feelings about yourself and the world.[5]

Then, within six months to a year, the majority of your excess weight falls off. You don't even completely realize that it's happening. You pass by a store window and stare at a reflection that for a couple of seconds you don't realize is actually you. You don't recognize yourself. You have the same hesitations about what chair to sit in, although, to your surprise, you now fit in all of them. You continue going to the large sizes' rack in the clothing department store, although you no longer need to.

LAWRENCE: *I remember going clothes shopping four months after the surgery. I used to be a 3x or 4x before, so I said to myself, "Well, I've lost some weight, so I'll start off with an extralarge." But it was too big. So I went and got a large. And I almost started to have a panic attack, physically. The large didn't fit, and so I went to get a medium. I tried it on, and it fit. And I just started crying in the dressing room because Lawrence doesn't wear a medium. It just doesn't happen!*

But something even more important is happening inside. You start changing the way you feel about yourself, about people, about your job, maybe even about your values. Who would have thought that losing weight could do this? Not too many of the people we interviewed expected it. And just about all of them expressed the feeling that they were always trying to catch up to the weight loss. They told us that changing the way they thought about themselves was in fact a lot harder and took a lot longer than losing the weight.

DAPHNE: *One of the things that I have noticed from having the surgery and the rapid weight loss is that, psychologically, you don't catch up to the physical changes. You see yourself shrinking, and you have to keep buying smaller clothes, and so you know the weight loss is happening. But psychologically the progress doesn't go at the same rate.*

This kind of disconnection between the physical self and the psychological self-concept can be quite a bizarre experience. You can now drop pounds from day to day, but how do you drop thirty years of learning, of thinking, of feeling? It's not that automatic.

DAPHNE: *I just haven't caught up psychologically. There are lots of things I can do now that I don't do. Why? Because in my head I still think I can't do them.*

The surgeon does not staple the brain. It may take years of unlearning to feel differently, and in some cases it may never happen, despite the smaller physique. Perhaps Erica put it best when she said, "The brain can hold on to the weight. The brain can mess with the laws of thermodynamics."

Chloe tried to explain to her new husband that she was not like any other 165-pound woman who had never been severely obese. She was a little more complicated. She came equipped with a bunch of fears and insecurities that no longer matched her body but were going to take some time to shake.

CHLOE: *"It's going to take time for me to understand that you see me as this person." I'm trying to believe that what's being said is truly about me and not about someone else.*

Chloe was having a hard time adapting to compliments and to sexual attention. She rejected them. She kept looking for the ulterior motive. She was doing the emotional equivalent of looking around the room to see who the compliment was really aimed at, because it could not possibly be her. This was disturbing to both her and her husband, who would never have guessed that complimenting his wife could possibly elicit suspicion or any kind of negative feelings. But it did, because the compliments did not match how Chloe saw herself. It made her wonder why he was saying things that, in her mind, could not possibly be true.

CHLOE: *It's still hard for me to see myself as a person of worth rather than as a liability. It's still hard. It's kind of new.*

For Penelope, the challenge manifested itself in an internal struggle between her old presurgical voice and her new postsurgical one. The old voice kept telling her that she could not do things—that she was not up to certain challenges. It wasn't a pleasant message, but it was a familiar one. She had spent a lifetime listening to that voice that stopped her from trying anything new. The postsurgical voice did the opposite. It spoke of all sorts of opportunities and urged her to push the envelope. She had to keep reminding herself which one to listen to.

PENELOPE: *Some of the confidence and self-esteem problems drag on—they hold on to you—but I'm slowly getting past it. It's the old script playing in your head. I ran into a couple of situations recently in which I realized that I was reacting like my old self and not like the new person. So I have to say, "Okay, let's put that voice on the side. Let's forget that doubting voice because that's the one that held you back, that's the one that made you feel bad about yourself." After a lifetime of not feeling confident, it's not something that's going to be cured in a day.*

From all accounts, listening to the new voice required practice. We don't get rid of lifelong patterns of thinking overnight. It takes a long time and a lot of work. Erica felt that it took her a long time to see herself differently after the surgery, and that it also took a long time for other folks to start seeing her as a "normal" person. Just as she continued to think she was fat even when she had lost almost half of her presurgical weight, she was pretty sure that other people continued to see her as fat long after she had lost the weight.

ERICA: *It takes a long time for your head to change and stop going to the size 24s when you walk into a store. It's also going to take a while for people around me to stop seeing me as that size 24.*

Having been obese seemed to have real sticking power. Some of our interviewees started wondering if it was something they would ever get over. Maybe the brain part of this surgery never really got "fixed." Weighing a mere 135 pounds ten years after the surgery, Maggie was still struggling to lose the presurgical ways of thinking and reacting.

MAGGIE: *There is still a part of me that says, "You can't." You end up believing all the negativity you experienced. You end up believing you can't accomplish anything. You should have been able to lose the weight without doing this, you should have taken pills or had your mouth wired or something . . . I lived with the "You should be able to. Can't you? Are you stupid?" I owned all of it, and it is still with me. I still fight it. And when somebody says, "You want to go and do such and such?" I still stop and think, "Do I want to?" Even when it is something I had always dreamed of doing.*

Maggie's difficulty in leaving the old defeatist self behind was clearly challenging to her. When she was obese she felt bad about being obese. When she had the surgery, she felt bad because she had not been able to accomplish the weight loss without resorting to such a radical intervention. She just couldn't shake the negativity completely—not yet. Even though it had been many years since she lost the weight, she continued to hesitate to agree to do things that she was actually yearning to do. That is a powerful testament to the staying power of old negative ways of thinking about ourselves and our lives. That's a whole ten years later!

Erica was not past the year mark when we interviewed her, but she was surprised that she had not yet lost the obese ways of thinking. One can only hope that it would not take as long for her as it was taking for Maggie.

ERICA: *I don't think I'm over being obese yet. It's still in my head in many ways. I'm still suffering from the effects of obesity, even though I'm not carrying the weight anymore. So, I'm not fully recovered. I'm beginning to think of it as being an alcoholic who will always have to go to* AA *[Alcoholics Anonymous].*

The comparison with alcoholism here is an interesting one. Although, as mentioned previously, it is controversial to consider eating an addiction, a lot of patients spoke of it that way. But here Erica is not talking about eating as an addiction—it's thinking like an obese person that she considers the addiction. What she can't shake is a specific way of thinking. The type of "AA" Erica needs is one that reminds her that she is no longer that heavy, that she no longer needs to anticipate negative reactions, that she is allowed to plan for and expect success here and there. The addiction she speaks of is an addiction to thinking negative thoughts.

The addiction analogy Erica chose to use may be a bit of a stretch, but it effectively communicates that obesity remained a state of mind for much longer than many of our interviewees had expected. From all accounts, that psychological transition was very difficult to accomplish.

MAGGIE: *I don't know whether there will ever be a time when I will see myself as thin. I don't know, but I still don't look in mirrors a whole lot. I didn't back then, and I still don't.*

One would think that with the dramatic weight loss, we would be rushing to a mirror for reinforcement, for evidence of success, at least once a day, if not more often. But that was not the case for Maggie. Mirrors were scary when she was obese, and they had not lost their power to terrify, even after her weight loss. She did not trust that she would be capable of seeing the weight loss in her reflection. She was afraid she would continue seeing herself as fat. After all, when she was obese she had not thought she looked *that* bad—

certainly not bad enough to do something about it. How would she know now if what she saw in the mirror was not just another distortion?

LAURA: *Years ago before I became obese, I saw myself as fat even when I was thin. Well, I finally became the fat person I always saw. I'm afraid I am always going to see myself as fat no matter how thin I get.*

Women with anorexia nervosa have perceptual distortions whereby they see themselves as fat when they are not.[6] It's not just that they want to be thin—it's that what they see in the mirror is much different from what other people see. Women with anorexia so severe they look like concentration-camp victims will tell you that what they see in the mirror is a fat girl. Our interviewees may have been suffering from similar perceptual distortions. When the interviewees were severely obese, their perception might have been that they weren't that fat. Now that they had lost a lot of weight, they looked in the mirror and still saw the fat person. Many surgery-seeking severely obese individuals meet some of the criteria for binge-eating disorder. It would thus not be surprising if clinically severe obesity shared some features with other eating disorders, such as distorted body image. In any case, mirrors remained unpredictable reference points after the surgery.

DAPHNE: *There are times when I look in the mirror and think, "Wow, you're looking good, girl! You got it going on!" Yet there are moments when I can look around, and I'm seeing the 350-pound girl again. And that gets to be depressing.*

The persistence of these old thought patterns was distressing for some folks. They wondered if they were ever going to feel good about themselves. Quincy also reported being unable to shake old patterns of behavior that had been organized around the obesity.

QUINCY: *I still don't talk to a lot of people because I still have it in the back of my head that I'm fat. So I don't talk. I listen.*

His self-consciousness when he was obese had made Quincy try to blend into the background, like wallpaper. If you don't talk, then no one will look at you and notice how big you are. He had done this when he weighed 444 pounds, but he was still doing it at 260. Ronald described the whole experience to us as follows: "It's like living in two worlds." You know intimately what it's like to live in the "fat" world. You've done it for decades. But now the surgery has given you access to this other world. Yet you cannot completely leave the world of your past, so you now feel like a tourist in both. You don't completely belong in either. You know what it's like to be obese, but you no longer are. You are now a person whose weight falls within norms, but you don't yet *know* how to be that. How does a person who is not obese feel and act?

QUINCY: *I don't think I'll ever get that feeling in my system of being completely positive because I was let down so many times because of my weight. I just take life as it is now.*

Does it ever change? Do you ever make it completely over to the thin side mentally and emotionally? Surely, many people do, but some of our interviewees had their doubts. They wondered if they would always be the outsiders, at least in their own minds. Not being considered an outsider by others was clearly not sufficient to make the transition. They needed to believe inside themselves that they were worthy. Being treated as such was great, but it was not enough. They needed to internalize these feelings of self-worth.

FRANCES: *I still feel like that large person on the inside. I kind of chuckle to myself that I can now pass. It makes me feel like a black person who could pass for a white person in the 1950s. You know, like being able to drink from the fountain, or sit in the front of the bus or something, but knowing you are still black. Well, I'm still that obese person you object to on the inside. I don't know if that ever changes. I've been told it's a process over time.*

The racial metaphor that Frances uses is a really powerful one here because it speaks to four important possibilities simultaneously:

1 that obesity is experienced, at least in part, as an essential quality that transcends weight and cannot be completely eliminated no matter how much weight is lost

2 that the world discriminates against obesity the way it discriminates against race

3 that just because right now you happen to be "passing," it does not mean the discrimination no longer exists—they just haven't noticed that you are not really "one of them"

4 that obese people internalize the discrimination similarly to the way other oppressed groups do

Living in a society that denigrates you cannot leave you unaffected. You may even subconsciously believe the negative stereotypes to some extent, even if you outwardly act as if you don't. Discrimination can be internalized even by the people being discriminated against. There is internalized sexism and racism and homophobia.[7] Some of our interviewees had clearly internalized "obesism," to make up a word here. Pretty powerful stuff! The shame of obesity proved very hard to get rid of, even if the obesity was now in the past. Brandon thought people's reluctance to tell others they had had the surgery was one manifestation of this shame.

BRANDON: *People say they don't want others to know they've had the surgery—that it's personal. But it's not the surgery they want to keep secret; it's the fact that they were once morbidly obese.*

The resilience of feeling obese surprised just about everyone we interviewed. Most had believed that the elimination of the fat would equal the elimination of their insecurities.

RONALD: *Things happen to me that help remind me that I am not big anymore, but in my own eyes, I'll always be big. Kind of like your kids will always be kids to you. Well, I'll always be big to me. I look in the mirror, and I don't see that much of a change when in fact I've lost 240 pounds!*

REX: *I still see myself as being overweight. I can't figure out when that's going to stop.*

Because of this haunting essence of obesity, a number of our interviewees shared the fantasy of escaping to a place where no one knew they had once been heavy. The dream was to make new friends and not tell them you were once obese, to move to a place where no one had known you back then. That would be one way of leaving the obesity behind. Or would it? The fantasy of leaving aspects of our lives behind by simply moving away or running in different social circles is a common one to many people for many reasons. The ability to reinvent ourselves and not be dogged by "old" perceptions of who we are is a fantasy we have all had at some point. When we were teenagers, we had fantasies of moving to a different high school where maybe we could lose the nicknames or unflattering social persona that had stuck to us. Maybe we could be cool somewhere else. It certainly wasn't going to happen in a place that had already decided we were uncool. Those things don't change easily. When we got older, maybe it was getting a new job in which we'd be the exciting new person instead of the unappreciated veteran. It's one of the attractions of leaving home when we are young, of going to college, of starting a new career in a new city, of dating someone new who hasn't already made up his mind about us. But what can we really leave behind? What is simply part of who we are, whether or not it is visible to others? These became essential questions for many of our interviewees.

GABRIELLE: *I have a new friend I've acquired in the last six or so months, and I don't want to tell her I was fat. Now, why is that important? I don't know. I don't want to forget the past, but in a sense I just want all of that to be over. I'm a thin person, so why does everyone have to know that I was a fat person?*

Gabrielle's question is an interesting one. Why was it *that* important that people not know they were once fat? One concern we already saw Erica express was the fear that people would continue to see you as an obese person with whatever attributes people attach to that. But in Gabrielle's case, she was even bothered by whether she should tell a new friend that she was ever fat at all. What did she fear her new friend would think? Did she fear she wouldn't respect her or be disappointed? Or could it be that, as Gabrielle said, she wanted to forget it *herself.* Telling her new friend would be a way of keeping one foot back in that fat world. In other words, is the fantasy of no one knowing you were obese rooted in a fear of judgment, or is it about your desire to escape your own assumptions of who you are or were? It's probably some combination of both of these motivations. Either way, a number of our interviewees thought wistfully about how nice it would be to start life over somewhere where no one knew they had once been obese.

> BRANDON: *It would be nice to lose all the weight but then relocate to a community where no one knew you before. Then people wouldn't have the stereotype or that image of me before I lost the weight.*

> ERICA: *I'm beginning to think about moving to a whole new city and start over to get away from this world that still sees me as fat. But I know I will still take this brain with me wherever I go, and I will continue to reach for the size 24 when I go to the store.*

Judging from many of the comments made, it seems unlikely that this fantasy of moving to another city would be that successful—that it would result in the total discarding of all aspects of the old obese self. Clearly, it was not just how people reacted that kept them stuck in the old self-concept. They carried it inside, and they would carry it to that new job, new relationship, or new city. It might help not to see the obese reflection of themselves in the eyes of people who knew them back then. On the other hand, it is unlikely that a move is all it would take to lose lifelong patterns of thinking, feeling, and perceiving. Despite Erica's frequent fantasies about moving away, she perhaps was the most eloquent in expressing how she would probably just carry the old way of thinking to wherever she ended up.

> ERICA: *Obesity is in my background, you know, like being from the Midwest. It will always be there.*

CHAPTER 5 | # Facing the Music of Self

When Weight Is No Longer the Reason

As you strip away the layers of fat,
you discover who you really are.
—MONA

Despite the tremendous growth in the popularity of obesity surgery in the past few years, it is still considered a relatively extreme intervention. It involves very direct surgical interference with our anatomy and physiology. It has significant risks and, depending on the type of surgery recommended (Lap-Band or gastric bypass or duodenal switch), it can be difficult, if not impossible, to reverse.[1] The very invasiveness of the procedure results in an interesting paradox. It's an extreme intervention typically reserved for extreme cases resulting in extreme outcomes. So why the big surprise when big changes happened? Why were most of our interviewees so shocked? Isn't that why they did it? Apparently, the extent and nature of the changes surpassed all expectations. It's almost as if the surgery itself were saying, "You wanted a big change? Well, you're going to get one! Fasten your seat belts!" And it was indeed a wild ride for many of the individuals we spoke to. Most expressed that they would do it again in a heartbeat, but they also seemed to be saying, "Be careful what you wish for" or maybe just "*Know* what you wish for." Their transitions were not always easy, but they involved an unexpected journey of personal growth that no one expressed a desire to reverse.

Immediately after the surgery, the weight started falling off at an incredibly quick rate. Six to eight months out of surgery, our interviewees had lost anywhere from 90 to more than 200 pounds. This is the honeymoon period in which many were deliriously happy with the amazing results. This surgery keeps its promise like few interventions do. A few months to a year into it, however, the weight loss started to slow down. The self-reflection and post-surgical questioning we discussed in the previous chapter started to make its way into their everyday thinking. They started realizing that this was about a lot more than weight. Somewhere between six months and a year after surgery, the honeymoon period was over. They were then faced with the fallout, good and bad, of the massive change they had undergone. They had arrived at their new destination, and, though most found it great and had no regrets, it was not always exactly as they thought it would be. In some cases, it was not even close. Things had happened to their lives they might never have believed had they been told beforehand. Or maybe having been told what *could* happen would have had a constructive impact in their coping with this unfamiliar postsurgical world.

> LAWRENCE: *The big thing that changed in my life . . . it was more of a mental thing. Six months after my surgery, I had lost all my weight. After that it was adjusting emotionally and mentally to what had happened. Those first few months are such a blur of activity, and you're excited because you're losing weight. Then, reality sets in.*

Some folks found that new reality easier than the old obese one on all fronts. Others found that each reality, the presurgical and the postsurgical one, held its own special set of challenges. Across the board, people reported a lot of personal growth as a function of the transition, along with significant growing pains. Insightful conclusions were not always easy to digest, so to speak, but they brought most of our interviewees closer to the truth of whom they were and who they really wanted to be.

What Made Me Fat in the First Place?

One of the unexpected consequences of the surgery was the personal search for the causes of the obesity. Everyone we interviewed had attended the same clinic and had been treated by the same doctor. Each had been required to attend a seminar on obesity and the details of the surgery prior to being evaluated as to their suitability for the procedure. That seminar reviewed the literature on clinically severe obesity comprehensively and emphasized the genetic contribution to the development of obesity. Yet as we mentioned in the last chapter, very few of our interviewees fell back on genetic explanations for their own obesity. This is in contrast to the common prejudice in the general population that obese people rationalize their condition with biological explanations that cover a weakness of character. There was little weakness of character evident in this group. The majority of our interviewees were deeply invested in discovering psychological and environmental factors that could explain how they had gotten that heavy in the first place. This issue became especially important because it involved the question of control. Although it may sometimes feel temporarily better to conclude that we've had no responsibility for a negative development in our lives, it also means we have no control. In the long run, the position of taking no responsibility is also the position of having no power. Our interviewees chose to cope with a little blame in order to gain a little control. If they could come to understand how they themselves had contributed to the obesity in the first place, then maybe they could make some changes to make sure they never let themselves get that obese again. Maybe this time they could be proactive.

LAWRENCE: *My obesity was related to emotional circumstances, and, you know, the surgery cannot cure your emotional state of mind. I was bored and I was depressed. Something was missing inside, and I was trying to feed that.*

Thirty-one years old and three years out of the surgery, Lawrence felt a pressing need to address his emotional problems because he feared that they might again lead him to obesity, despite the surgery. That would feel truly inexcusable to him. Considering that a significant number of people who have undergone weight loss surgery do regain the weight when they fail to adhere to the required dietary regimen, Lawrence's concern was not unfounded. That three-year mark was a dangerous time. He had reached his target weight of 160 after the surgery, but at the time of the interview, he was 10 pounds heavier. That seemed like nothing compared to his presurgical weight of 330, but that is how it starts when people regain. A pound here, a pound there, and suddenly it's out of control again. Maladaptive eating patterns such as grazing, making poor food choices, eating in response to negative emotions, and even eating too much at each setting could all contribute to weight regain (see C. G. Fairburn's *Overcoming Binge Eating* in the Appendix for help with this problem). The surgery does nothing to get rid of your desire to eat and whatever role food played in your life. Echoing Lawrence, Maggie said, "The surgery doesn't cure what made you heavy in the first place." And many of our interviewees felt that emotional issues were at the bottom of things.

For individuals who engaged in emotional eating (eating as an attempt to escape negative emotions), figuring this out was crucial.[2] Maggie knew she had "turned to food for comfort—as something to hide behind." Emotional eating was no longer an option, yet there was so much emotion floating around because of all of the postsurgical challenges. Our interviewees' lives were changing in good, but sometimes scary, ways. Maybe they were dating for the first time or their established relationships were shifting on them. Maybe they were facing new professional opportunities with all the anxiety that they can create. Since the weight loss, excuses for saying no to new experiences had evaporated, and our interviewees were no longer shielded from all the emotion that goes with these new experiences. For many, the emotion was running even higher than it had been when they were obese. So paradoxically, the surgery had in some ways exacerbated the psychological conditions that had traditionally led them to eat. But now, eating could not be a viable method of self-soothing if they were going to lose the weight and keep it off. Food could no longer be used as a vehicle to anxiety reduction. Food could no longer rescue them from what they were feeling.

> MAGGIE: *I now have to deal with problems that I always fed with my addiction to food. Sometimes I don't really want to have to deal with these problems. It was much easier to just shove them to the side, pat them down, and cover them with food and move on to something else.*

Frances wondered if severe obesity, much like the recognized eating disorders, was not a reaction to societal pressures to look a certain way, to be thin and beautiful as conventionally defined.

FRANCES: *Even thin women feel bad about themselves. It's kind of a chicken-or-egg thing—could it be that feeling so negatively about yourself could result in morbid obesity and not just anorexia? As a form of protection against the pressure?*

It's an interesting idea that the societal pressure to be thin might lead to one of two extreme reactions: starvation to hyperconform to the beauty ideal or overeating to either rebel against the ideal or maybe just give up entirely on ever attaining it. But why would these media and societal messages of inadequacy not lead everyone to an eating disorder, and why would it lead some women to overeat and others to undereat? These are all very important questions that science is working hard to tease apart. The answers appear to be quite complex and involve factors from three different dimensions: biology, psychology, and social forces. All women in Western society are exposed, more or less, to the same pressures to attain an ideal of beauty that is unrealistic. Since these social forces are ubiquitous and all Western women are equally exposed to them, the explanation for eating-disordered behavior cannot just lie in social pressures, or else all women would have eating disorders. The truth is that the prevalence rates for each of the eating disorders remains relatively low. The number of late-adolescent and adult women in the United States who will meet the full criteria for a diagnosis of anorexia nervosa in their lifetime is approximately 0.5 to 3.7 percent of the population, and for bulimia nervosa it is about 1.1 to 4.2 percent. Between two and three out of every one hundred American men and women will experience binge-eating disorder in a six-month period.[3] That would still leave approximately 90 percent of all the women who are exposed to the very same societal messages about the thinness ideal without an eating disorder. Although many of these women may still feel negatively about their bodies, with most of them either on a diet or contemplating one, very few develop eating disorders. So there must be something different about women who fall prey to disordered-eating behavior. This something special could be a biological predisposition, or it could be a personality trait given to behavioral extremes. For example, Maggie was pretty sure she became obese because of a personality characteristic. Ten years out of surgery, she was still fighting against the recommended diet.

> MAGGIE: *I have a very compulsive personality, and I push everything to the limit. I still experiment to see what I can get away with foodwise. It's not the best thing to do, but it's my personality, and it always comes out. If you tell me I shouldn't do something, I'm going to try it just to see whether it can be done or not.*

This trait made Maggie push the envelope even after the surgery. She was worried about her propensity to try to eat more than she should or to eat things she shouldn't just to see if she could get away with it. Obviously, this is a dangerous attitude that could easily lead to weight regain. Clearly, the surgery had not done much to change that vulnerability, and unless Maggie made extraordinary efforts to keep that side of her personality in check, it could lead right back to where she started—clinically severe obesity.

A couple of women in our group placed the blame for their obesity squarely on the shoulders of childhood sexual abuse. They believed that they had started to gain weight to desexualize themselves—if they were fat, then maybe no one would approach them sexually. This explanation made them doubly frightened by the prospect of losing the weight and again entering the realm of male-female relationships.

> LAURA: *I have something on my forehead. It started when I was three years old, and it only stopped when I got fat. Men screw me. I was molested by everyone and their dog the whole time I was growing up. I have also been raped. So I say to myself, "It can't just be them!" So I'm scared. I want to be thin so bad. I want people to notice me. I want people to see me, but I'm so scared that somehow . . . If it happens again, I just can't . . .*

It is noteworthy that Laura believes she is somehow marked, that the trauma she experienced in her life has something to do with who she is, what she communicated, even at the age of three! It is not unusual for victims of sexual abuse and assault to feel guilty and blame themselves, especially if they are women.[4] This is not surprising considering that, for decades, women who were sexually traumatized were openly blamed for it, even by the justice system. These malicious attributions are often internalized by the victims, just as ethnoracial groups can internalize racism and gays and lesbians can internalize homophobia. In many other cultures, women are still blamed for "bringing on" the sexual assaults. The "blaming the victim" strategy is as old as the hills and effective for those who seek to hold on to their power over women. On the other hand, it is probably healthy for Laura to think about what she can do to make as sure as she can that it never happens to her again. Often, women who have experienced sexual abuse have their judgment about men and certain situations damaged in the process. Without assigning one bit of blame to them, it is sometimes critical for them to review their judgment about risk and circumstance. Their radar for danger and their radar for real love rather than objectification can be broken. Working to improve their judgment can be all about taking their power back. After all, for someone like Laura, the development of good judgment about men and relationships would be critical. If she, in fact, gained the weight consciously or subconsciously to desexualize herself and escape the threatening world of sexuality, then it would be essential that her weight loss *not* result in a return to abusive relationships. If it did, there would be a pretty good chance that Laura would gain her weight back, going from danger right back to safety.

And so, our interviewees explained how they become severely obese in a number of ways:

- emptiness, depression, and negative emotion

- a propensity to use eating as a way of coping with emotion, as a way of self-soothing

- rebellion against societal pressure to attain an unattainable body ideal

- a personality-based tendency toward extreme behavior

- an attempt to desexualize oneself after sexual trauma or abuse

Some of the explanations were situational, whereas some were personality-based. Most of our interviewees had been severely obese for so long that they couldn't be completely confident about their assessments of what came first—the obesity or the negative emotions. As Frances said, trying to figure it out had a bit of the "chicken or the egg" dilemma, but most thought it was useful to try to tease apart cause and effect. By engaging in this self-reflective exercise, they were hoping to raise their level of awareness about their feelings and behaviors. They hoped it would keep them from sleepwalking back to that terrible place.

Losing the Armor of Fat

It may seem counterintuitive to think about severe obesity as protective. After all, this very obesity had made many of our interviewees the butt of jokes and mockery in a society cruelly unforgiving of departures from the conventional aesthetic. They all gave vivid examples of the way in which obesity had made them victims of humiliation, hostility, and neglect. There is little doubt that obesity had in fact invited many attacks of this sort. But, interestingly, it had also protected them against other challenges. Perhaps the biggest of these challenges had been an accurate appraisal of their capabilities and even of their own personalities. While obese, they could blame their failures on the weight and thus never really discover whether this explanation was true. If someone didn't like them, it was because they were fat. If they didn't get that promotion, it was because they were fat. If they didn't have friends, it was because they were fat. If they couldn't get a date, it was because they were fat. Now the weight was off, and those attributions were being put to the test. And that was scary! What if they'd been wrong in blaming the weight, at least sometimes? What if the reason some of these things had or hadn't happened lay in their personalities or abilities and not in the number of pounds on the scale and the accompanying discrimination?

LAURA: *I put all my goals on hold until I lost the weight. "Okay, I'm going to be this great singer when I lose the weight." I had the same voice then, but everything was about after I lose the weight, after I lose the weight. Now that the weight is coming off, it's like, "Uh oh! Oh, crap, can I really do this? I am not huge anymore. I really could go up and do this now." And I am trying. But I have a real fear of being rejected for who I really am and not just because I am a fat person.*

It is extremely difficult for anyone to make it as a singer. Laura was probably correct in thinking that it was going to be particularly challenging to succeed while obese. Although there are some singers who overcame that handicap, such as Aretha Franklin and Barry White to name just two, there is little question that the industry continues to be largely driven by looks, especially in regard to women. So Laura was not entirely deluded in thinking her weight might get in the way. The problem, however, was that she could also use the obesity as an excuse for not trying. Alternately, even if she tried really hard to succeed and still didn't make it, Laura would never know if her weight was the reason she had failed. However, she could always blame the weight to make herself feel better either for not trying or for not making it. It could be a self-esteem-saving explanation. And there's nothing inherently wrong with esteem-saving attributions unless, of course, they are keeping us from accomplishing our goals and being truly content.

ERICA: *There's lots of benefits to being fat. They are sick benefits, but they are benefits. I think I have finally gotten to the point in my life in which I can face that if I fail, it is because of me and not because of my fat.*

It's not hard to see why it would be difficult to get to that point. Facing the truth is not always easy. We all struggle to discover the reasons for our failures. Sometimes we internalize and blame ourselves. More often, though, we look outward and lay it at somebody else's door. "I didn't get the job because he didn't like me, or because I threatened him, or because I am a woman, or because I am Latina." Sometimes these attributions are true. Life can be unfair, and we can be denied what we deserve for arbitrary or discriminatory reasons well outside of our control. However, there is something we might be well advised to red-flag. If the explanations we come up with are more often than not ones that place the responsibility on others rather than ourselves, then we are probably not being honest with ourselves. There is a pretty good chance that we are engaging in esteem-saving strategies that ultimately interfere with personal growth. Rather than working at self-improvement, we may be simply externalizing all failures (it's always somebody else's fault). "I'm where I need to be—it's them who have it all wrong. Simon and Paula and Randy are deaf or crazy—they don't realize that I am the next American idol!"

MONA: *You know being fat is a huge gimme. It's a big, fat cop-out! And now I don't have that big, fat cop-out anymore because some people are still rejecting me as a thin person. "Hey, wait a minute! You're not supposed to be rejecting me when I'm thin. You were supposed to be rejecting me when I was fat. But damn it, now I'm thin so the world should be my oyster, and I should be able to have it all."*

We all engage in the creation of stories (narratives) that make us feel better about ourselves. Some of these narratives are mostly true, some are probably fifty-fifty, and others are likely to be mostly false. We might think, "Who cares if the stories are accurate, if they make us feel better?" This is the "whatever gets you through the night" approach, and there is some logic to it. However, false self-narratives have consequences. As already mentioned above, they promote stasis (lack of growth), and they block self-improvement. But they are even more harmful than that. They are likely to play havoc on our relationships, at work, at play, and at home. After all, we may have convinced ourselves of our esteem-saving narrative, but convincing others is a whole other story. They are not as motivated as we are to buy our self-enhancing explanations. They will more likely see the falsehood in our story and judge us for it. In addition, if we have a tendency to blame others for our failures, those others will get angry by what they feel is an unfair accusation. Striving for accuracy rather than self-soothing in our stories about what caused what is very difficult, but it is likely to take us to a better place both personally and interpersonally.

If Laura does in fact give her singing career all she's got, it could get her a recording contract or not. If the outcome is not successful, it will be disappointing, but she will know that she did her best and that a singing career was simply not in the cards for her. Which is better, to think she never got that recording contract because she was fat or because she simply wasn't good enough? Laura would have to answer that for herself. The bottom line, however, is that the "I can't succeed because I am fat" strategy is a sure bet—she won't try, so there will be no record contract. The "going for it" strategy at least has a chance of success. It's just that it also carries a risk—the risk of discovering that maybe she is not sufficiently talented. The point is that our self-worth is best placed within what we can control—in the quality of our efforts rather than in the outcome. Easier said than done for all of us, no doubt!

Lawrence recounted an actual failure after the weight loss that drove the point home for him in no uncertain terms.

> LAWRENCE: *For instance, if I didn't get hired for a job, I could always say it was because I was fat. If I didn't accomplish something, it was because I was fat. And then when I had lost the weight, something happened to me. I did not pass an important practical-skills exam. And it was funny because the first thing that jumped into my mind was, "Oh, they failed me because I am fat." And then suddenly I said to myself, "Whoa, wait a second. I'm not fat. They didn't do anything." That just floored me. That was the first slap in the face.*

Lawrence's automatic response to his failure had been to blame it on the weight. It was what he had typically done over a lifetime of obesity. Suddenly, he realized that the explanation no longer worked. He was so accustomed to blaming failure on the weight that he had momentarily forgotten that he was not heavy anymore. The excuse had dissolved along with his lipid levels. For the first time, he saw the role that obesity had played as an esteem-saving narrative. But, in fact, the narrative had carried a double danger. As in the case of Laura, it had kept Lawrence from the truth of his abilities, whatever they were, in any given situation. In addition, it had also created a feeling of resentment for others that at times may have been completely undeserved.

So the armor of fat had "protected" him from painful self-realizations, yet it had also created a feeling of hostility toward people who may have done nothing to engender it.

When you start looking closely at the kind of "protection" that the obesity afforded our interviewees, it does not sound very protective at all—as a matter of fact, it seems quite destructive. Protecting ourselves from truthful self-revelations works directly against personal progress and self-improvement. Attributing failures to others or circumstances may feel momentarily satisfying in one sense, but it also negates our control and mastery over the world. Saying "It's not us but them" also means that we are unlikely to engage in any attempts to get better at whatever it is we do. With no sense of agency, what's the point in trying? We believe it is out of our hands. It also produces a siege mentality in which the world is our enemy. This is poison to relationships. It is impossible to have successful relationships without owning a part of both the joy and the pain. If weight becomes the standard reason we give ourselves for every interpersonal failure, then it is unlikely that we are going to develop lasting relationships. Why? For one, we will feel constantly slighted by almost everyone. We will create for ourselves the paranoid illusion that everyone is discriminating against us. This just simply is unlikely to be true, yet in so believing it, we rob ourselves of potentially gratifying relationships.

CHLOE: *When I was fat, I would not allow anyone to love me. That was my wall, my protection. I wouldn't let people in.*

In this siege mentality, we also fail to learn how to correct our own behavior because we are not reality testing—we aren't asking friends and family what they think about how we acted because we don't trust anyone. And this is an important function of relationships, as, even with the best intentions, we have all engaged in behavior that is interpersonally injurious. We need to be able to listen to our friends when they tell us that something we did might not have been very nice. So . . . so much for the protection of fat! It might have protected in some ways, but the price was the following:

⊙ reduced self-awareness and self-knowledge

⊙ reduced sense of control and agency

⊙ distrust of others

⊙ hostility toward others

⊙ social isolation

⊙ little reality testing about our feelings and behavior

⊙ enhanced likelihood that we will engage in interpersonally hurtful behavior

Better to leave that and any other hugely self-deceptive shield by the wayside. It is ultimately not a pleasant way to live for most people.

Furthermore, do we really 100 percent believe our not-so-true stories about ourselves? Maybe some people do, but many of us admit to having some doubts about the reasons we give ourselves for why it was "them" and not us. We are often left with a nagging feeling that maybe, just maybe, we did something to contribute to the undesired situation. Essentially, most well-adjusted people are not completely successful in the art of self-deception. We probably spend more time and energy than we would like to admit pushing back the doubts about our responsibility in any given situation. And one has to wonder if that is time and energy well spent.

Yet facing the world those first few months after surgery without the "protection" of obesity can be very difficult. Lawrence had quite vividly ex-pressed that his first brush with failure after the weight loss was a "slap in the face." Self-discovery is challenging, even if it eventually leads to a posi-tive outcome. It's one of those processes that feels worse before it feels bet-ter. It involves looking coldly at ourselves and identifying those aspects that we would like to change. Prior to succeeding in the change, all we have is the not-so-pleasant realization of our weaknesses. Many of our interviewees found it the singularly most difficult aspect of the weight loss.

ERICA: *The hardest thing about the surgery is that you realize you were blaming all your problems on your weight and then when you lose the*

weight and realize the problems weren't all weight related. I don't just
blame myself for the fact that I had expectations about the ways in which
weight loss was going to change my life. I also blame society, which has
always told you that you could do so much if you lost weight. You know,
"You are such a beautiful woman, and if you just lost weight . . ."

Clearly, Erica did not just blame herself for the deceptive narrative about weight being the only barrier to success. She thought society had played a major role in the development of that narrative. And she was not wrong. We most certainly live in a society that places an extremely high premium on conventional concepts of beauty, especially for women. The media bombard us with messages about how true happiness is just outside our reach—attainable only through the latest beauty product, exercise machine, fad diet, or cosmetic procedure. Most of us fall victim to that message in some form or another. Listen for long enough to one of those infomercials about a product that takes five inches off your waistline or ten years off your face in a month, and soon enough you are considering making that phone call. The implication is that those five inches or ten years are standing between you and fulfillment. We have also all seen those makeover shows in which women are transformed before our very eyes into supposed beauties. They are implying that the true path to happiness is physical beauty. The mental and emotional stuff is beside the point! So Erica was hearing people say to her that she was a beautiful woman who was hampered only by weight. The message was clearly "Lose the weight and the beauty will rise to the surface, and you will live happily ever after." Not that simple, apparently. And Erica was partly justified in pointing a finger at a world that supports and reinforces this deceptive narrative about the attainment of happiness. Unfortunately for Erica, she felt she had not gotten very far in her pursuit of the life she had dreamed of. She felt betrayed by the implied promise of weight loss.

ERICA: *I want what I've never had, and the whole world has always told*
me that if I lost the weight I would get it, and I'm angry that is has not
come. There will always be a certain level of dissatisfaction in my life. I
still have it, and I've added a couple of pockets of anger that I didn't have
before because of this new situation and its disappointments.

Doris was also very disappointed, but, unlike Erica, she blamed herself mostly. Her inability to find happiness after surgery suggested to her that maybe she just had a predisposition to find the one negative aspect of every circumstance, the opposite of wearing rose-colored glasses.

DORIS: *Today I was in my bedroom crying. I hated myself when I was fat, I still feel fat, and if I ever get truly skinny, I'm going to be tripping over my tits—am I ever going to feel satisfied?*

Doris is asking herself a very good question here. Will she ever be happy? She is starting to wonder. As she is experiencing the weight loss she had always longed for, her happiness level has not risen substantially. And when she thinks ahead to when she will attain her target weight, she worries that she'll still be unhappy because of her sagging breasts. This raises the whole issue of happiness and the extent to which any one individual can feel it. Much research now confirms that by the time we are adults, we seem to have a predisposition toward a certain level of happiness, barring traumatic experiences.[5] This predisposition for happiness is not unlike the idea that we may have a predisposition toward a specific weight. Some researchers believe that there is a certain weight that our bodies tend to gravitate toward unless we do something relatively drastic. They call this a set point for weight, although this theory is not without controversy.[6] Well, just like we may have individual set points for weight, we may have individual set points for happiness. A number of studies have shown that the happiness levels of most individuals change only *very temporarily* when either something very positive or something very negative happens.[7] Lottery winners tend to revert back to their usual levels of happiness once the initial euphoria wears off. The same is true for individuals who have just received a diagnosis of HIV infection. After the initial shock and grief, they also revert back to their regular happiness set point. Yet none of us really truly believes these findings until we experience them. Many of us are convinced that we would stay elated if we suddenly became millionaires and that we would stay depressed if we suddenly got a diagnosis of a chronic and debilitating illness. But the data suggest that we are wrong. It is interesting to see how this plays out in the context of obesity surgery.

Doris had fallen into the trap of thinking that the weight loss (like the lottery) would finally bring her the happiness that had eluded her. But maybe Doris does not have a big capacity for happiness. Maybe she will always struggle to maintain positive affect. There is, however, something very hopeful in Doris even asking herself the question about whether she will ever be happy. It means that she is finally considering the fact that the major obstacle to her happiness may lie in her overall outlook rather than in the weight or the sagging skin or whatever else may follow. If she figures that out, she may be able to work on her predisposition toward negativity and find some satisfaction in her life.

Even Erica, angry and disappointed though she feels about the failed promise of a better life after weight loss, knows that responsibility for her happiness lies in her brain and not in her girth.

ERICA: *I'm facing reality. I had to get to a point at which I did not need the weight psychologically as much. I didn't hide behind it anymore. But I still need to lose more weight, and I've stopped losing for now. My honeymoon period [when the weight comes off relatively effortlessly] was pretty short. I think that's because I still need the weight. When I get my head straight, the rest will go. When I get my head on square, my body will be thin.*

Nine months after surgery, Erica had dropped from 350 pounds to 205, but the weight had stopped falling off effortlessly. Erica continued to adhere to the diet, so she convinced herself that the reason she had stopped losing was psychological. She actually thought she was holding on to the weight with her mind. It is hard to know exactly how she thought her mind was accomplishing that, but what is important is that Erica was acknowledging the protective role of weight and taking responsibility for holding on to it. We hope that Erica lost her need for the weight and that this was accompanied by a corresponding satisfaction and happiness that had not yet materialized at the time of our interview.

The fantasy that life will be perfect after the weight loss is also propped up by the self-defeatism of the severely obese person. Most severely obese people have lost all hope that they will ever lose the weight. In a sense, this attitude makes it easier to imagine the perfection of a thin life. It's like a fairy tale you can tell yourself. You don't ever expect to have to witness whether the frog ever becomes the prince or Cinderella ever escapes her evil step-mother's grasp. You can safely assume it, because you don't believe you will ever be in a position to put it to the test.

FRANCES: *Since part of me thought I would never lose the weight, I could have the fantasy that if I were thin, then no negative things would be happening. Everything would just be perfect.*

The journey from that "first slap in the face" to a more developed self-discovery and positive change was not easy. However, a number of our interviewees believed they had navigated it successfully and came out feeling much better at the other end. "Convenient" excuses for failures were recognized for the burden they actually were, the ball and chain that kept them from the freedom of exploring all of their potential. A couple of our interviewees were even happy to lose the excuse of weight as a reason to magnify presurgical successes. Both failures and successes had now become just that and nothing more. The weight finally had nothing to do with anything!

FRANCES: *Weight is a nonissue for me now. It is no longer a way to excuse my failures or to make my successes even more meaningful. It is so liberating not to have to live that way anymore. It was the reason I didn't get asked out, it was the reason I didn't get the job I wanted, it was the excuse I used for everything.*

The loss of excuses as a move toward liberation and growth was also echoed by Lawrence.

LAWRENCE: *Getting my life back on track has been a challenge because I had to confront my individual issues. For example, I was really unhappy at my job. Really unhappy. I just never had the courage to change it. Being fat was a good excuse not to change jobs. And finally I got the courage to quit my job and go back to school. That represents a 75 percent pay cut, but I'm going to be doing something that I want to be doing!*

The road from the protection against failure to the striving for our dreams looks like a pretty positive trajectory. Most people's dreams are perfectly attainable. Laura's dream to be a successful singer was a big one, and she may or may not become the next vocal sensation, but there were probably many second-order dreams in her bag that she was pretty much assured to reach if she just tried. And that is true for most of the dreams that our obese folks had. The fat wasn't protecting them from delusional dreams about being president or a rock star or a Nobel laureate. The fat was "protecting" them against better jobs, pursuing a higher education, having a relationship—all things within reach for most people as long as they reach out to get them. The feeling of hope pervaded most of their stories of struggle toward these goals.

HELENA: *There is nothing so bad that I can't deal with it. I can deal with anything because the worst thing in my life was obesity, and I dealt with that. So, I can deal with other minor stumbling blocks that may fall in my path.*

Owning What's Yours

Once the weight was no longer an available alibi, folks had to face up to what they owned. Lawrence, for one, found that to be a substantial challenge.

LAWRENCE: *Realizing that the problems in my life were not all weight-related was a big change emotionally.*

Now they had to come to terms with their strengths and weaknesses, weight issues aside. It was difficult and it was exhilarating. It was liberating and it was depressing. It was essentially what each individual decided it was going to be. Nobody seemed entirely prepared for this part of the journey.

FRANCES: *Some of the problems I was prepared for. I think I knew at some level I would have to face them, and I was prepared to deal with them. But some totally blindsided me.*

Most folks, however, seemed up to the challenge. Whether the news was good or bad, most people seemed to face head-on whatever their new life said about who they were.

> URSULA: *You have to take a look at yourself and sometimes that's really hard, and sometimes it's not much fun to look at what's making you do what you do and act in the way you act. You have to be psychologically ready for this surgery because it forces you to look inside yourself, and that can be very hard.*

For Daphne, facing her "real" self and her non-weight-related problems was in some ways as challenging as it had been to admit that she was severely obese prior to the surgery.

> DAPHNE: *It's like admitting that you are a fat person. You know it's humiliating, so you don't confront it. You act as if the problem doesn't exist. In the back of your mind, you know it's there, but you don't confront it and the problem never gets addressed. That's the problem with most obese people. Who wants to admit they have a problem?*

Daphne is here making the point that, hard as it is for anyone to admit that they have a problem, it might even be a little harder for people with a history of obesity. In her estimation, that very history of obesity was proof that obese individuals are a group particularly adept at denial.

Arriving at the realization that not all of life's problems disappeared with the weight also brought about a quasi reconciliation with the "thin world." Before the surgery, some of our interviewees thought that misery belonged to the obese and that, somehow, the nonobese enjoyed a carefree life that in no way resembled theirs. This falls somewhere into the "grass is always greener on the other side" conclusion that we are all so subject to. The realization that life was challenging even without the weight brought about a feeling of fraternity with nonobese people, one that had not existed during the obese years. It increased empathy for others, and it erased that partly false dividing line.

FRANCES: *Thin people have problems too. I have simply traded the problems I had when I was obese, like not fitting into an airplane seat, for a new set of problems I had never dealt with.*

ERICA: *It's not all wonderful after the surgery. It's still life. Society tells us that our problems are caused by our weight, and they are not.*

Suddenly, it became apparent that thin people had problems also. They were just different and not necessarily any easier—simply different. There was a general feeling among our interviewees that they had traded one set of problems for a completely different set. Maybe now they were not worrying about managing their diabetes or fitting into restaurant booths or embarrassing their children. But now they had to learn how to deal with their spouses' mounting insecurities, or wonder why they did not get that promotion since they could no longer blame the weight. These were new dilemmas, and they were not easy to figure out. And those new issues were simply piled on to the old problems they had never expected the surgery to resolve.

HELENA: *Some people think this is the perfect cure-all for everything in their lives. But it's not. You swap one set of issues for another set of issues. And you just have to deal with the swapping of the issues and that it's not a big deal. Losing weight does not make the world perfect. There are still going to be wars and interest rates and the husband and kids with the mortgage and car payments.*

Some folks quickly realized that the problems they had before the surgery were going to persist. Changing them would require a different kind of intervention—one that did not involve a scalpel.

ERICA: *The surgery affected me physically, but I've got the same demons I had before. I guess I was blaming most of the problems in my life on my obesity beforehand, and now I'm coming to the realization that it's really me, not the weight. I haven't gotten a better job, and I haven't fallen in love and lived happily ever after.*

As we have seen before, Erica felt pretty down about the whole thing. She had not yet found a way to deal with her demons, and she remained stuck in feelings of anger and disappointment. Frances and Karina, on the other hand, found the whole thing difficult but liberating.

> FRANCES: *Losing the weight means that I can fail and succeed on my own terms without always tagging the weight as the reason something did or did not happen. But it's also frightening because I can't blame the weight anymore. I have to say, "Well, maybe I'm just not good at this, or maybe they just don't like me." Before I was always able to believe that if I was thin, things would have worked out.*

> KARINA: *For the first time in my life I have control. It's up to me whether I succeed or fail.*

Irma was able to look coldly at the reality of a recent failure to get a promotion and felt perfectly at peace dealing with what she considered to be the truth of it. She was happy to be able to face it and feel fine. She was happy to no longer have the weight to blame.

> IRMA: *A couple of years ago I tried out for a promotion, and I know I didn't get it because I was fat. I know I was qualified for it. This last one, I knew I wasn't as qualified for. Whether I was 250 pounds or 150 pounds, I didn't get it because I wasn't qualified for it, but had I weighed 250 when I got turned down, I would have thought it was because I was obese.*

Perhaps one of the healthiest developments that accompanied the dissolution of the armor of fat was a growing sense of self-acceptance. Although we have spoken much in this chapter about striving and trying to be the best that you can be, it is equally important to accurately assess our limitations and find a sense of self-worth despite our deficits. We do not all have the same level of abilities in all arenas. We will succeed in some and fail in others, and that is absolutely everybody's truth, without exception. Failure does not indicate worthlessness. It is an integral part of being alive.

> FRANCES: *Before, the thought of failing was the worst thing. Now the knowledge that I'm not going to be good at everything and that by the law of averages I'm not going to succeed at everything is okay.*

Although she struggled with feelings of negativity, Erica was also working on developing a greater acceptance of herself.

> ERICA: *People hit their forties, and they get past the era of high expectations. They stop expecting to be president or the top of their field. I guess that's where I am now—I am more accepting of who Erica is these days.*

This acceptance was integral for our interviewees. They had lived a life of rejection. They had blamed themselves and been blamed by others for their obesity. This had had the effect of making them either withdraw from society and themselves or make superhuman attempts to prove their worth to self and others. It was time to give themselves a bit of a break. It was time to let themselves be who they really were without harsh judgments raining down.

Is There a User's Manual to the New Me?

The problems of being clinically severely obese were many, and they were very significant, from not being able to take a walk without being out of breath to being ridiculed, judged, and stuck at home wondering if you would ever have a significant love affair or wondering if you were going to die in your sleep. These problems were painful enough for folks to opt for this difficult and invasive surgery. Yet these problems had become familiar over the years. Many of the people we interviewed had close to a lifetime's practice in dealing with the problems of severe obesity. To some extent, they had learned how to ignore the stares of others, they had learned to dismiss other people's judgments, and they had almost convinced themselves that maybe that love affair was not that important anyway. Fortunately, their ways of coping had not been all that successful or they would not have had the surgery, but they had their techniques for dealing with old, familiar problems. The weight loss, however, presented them with a new set of challenges they had no idea how to cope with. They had had no practice whatsoever with certain kinds of problems.

FRANCES: *When you have the surgery, the armor disappears, and you are not prepared to fight fights you never had to fight before because the weight was a shield.*

For some individuals, the loss of the armor and the challenges of a whole new set of life circumstances made them feel extremely vulnerable and exposed. The weight really had acted as a cover under which to hide. This sounds like a nice metaphor, but some of our interviewees were not being poetic when they talked about the fat as a hiding place or an armor. They quite literally experienced the weight loss as a shocking exposure—almost as if they suddenly found themselves naked in public.

MONA: *I am going through a "midfat crisis." Without all the excuses, you are vulnerable. I feel so vulnerable, so out there.*

Mona's description of her state as a "midfat crisis" is very evocative. We are all familiar with the concept of a midlife crisis in which one feels panic at the realization of advancing age while still feeling young and attached to the lifestyle of our youth. It is a difficult transition for a lot of people and a pretty good analogy for the experience of some of our interviewees. In her "midfat crisis," Mona felt stuck in the strange netherland between her obese self and her new thin one. She was still attached to familiar ways of thinking and behaving, yet she felt this huge change in her body. This change was presenting her with both emotional and behavioral challenges she did not yet know exactly how to deal with. The new self-realizations were shocking enough, but now she also had to learn to deal with people—people who had avoided her and whom she had avoided for a good part of her life.

MAGGIE: *I hid behind my wall of fat and didn't want to deal with people. It hurt because I knew people didn't want to deal with me, and the fat was my way of not having to deal with them. And then all of a sudden I lost the weight, and I ran into people who knew I had been heavy and people who didn't, and they all treated me so differently. They ignored me before and now they didn't, and that kicked in a whole new set of problems, like*

not being resentful about that, like learning to deal with different indi-
viduals and their feelings about me. So for a while I had the old problems
to deal with and these new ones also. And so consequently, it was an ex-
tremely hard adjustment.

Difficulty being social was a very common report among our interviewees. Obesity had been an isolating experience. The world rejected the obese,
and the obese rejected the world. Better not to want what doesn't want you
than to live in an unrequited state of desire. Avoiding people had come natu-
rally to many. What was the point of social contact? You risked feeling embarrassed, judged, ignored, or used. People could not be trusted to treat you
right. It may have been a lonely life for many, but preferable to the threat of
getting hurt. Suddenly, with the weight loss, the social world came knocking,
and many of our interviewees had a hard time trusting the new attention.

MAGGIE: *The weight loss has created a lot of situations that I still don't*
want to deal with as far as human-to-human contact. I have a hard time
with that, being intimate, trusting people.

The development of mistrust in relationships is not eradicated overnight.
For many, the weight was gone well before they had relearned to trust people. Letting people in continued to feel dangerous. And there was also the
problem of a missing skill set. After so many years of avoiding social contact,
some of our interviewees did not know how to be with people, how to act,
what to say. It was all new.

URSULA: *I used my weight as protection against the outside world.*
Maybe this had something to do with the abuse I experienced as a child.
The bigger I got, the more personal space I felt I had. So when I lost the
weight, that protection was gone, and people wanted to get into my space.
It is still difficult for me to let people get close to me. It's a real conflict that
I fight every day. Aarghhh! It's just real hard to accept the fact that it's okay
to let people in.

Some folks had dealt with the rejection by being openly hostile to other
people. Their defense had clearly been to attack. That way, when people re-

jected you, you knew why—because you had not been nice to them. That had felt easier than being rejected simply because of the way you look. For those who had defended themselves with this tactic, the challenge became to learn to be nice to people. For Quincy, that was also a new skill set he had to work hard to acquire.

QUINCY: *I'm afraid I'm going to say the wrong thing and hurt people.*

With the weight loss, Quincy finally acknowledged that he wanted the care and approval of others. However, he had spent so many years being ornery that he wasn't sure how to be nice, and he was afraid he'd turn people off—something he'd almost taken pride in when he was very heavy.

Other folks had problems getting used to their new bodies. They did not recognize its bumps and curves and even feared that something was wrong with this new body.

KARINA: *I'll be laying in bed, and I'll say to my husband, "Do I have a bump here? What is that?" And he'll say, "Ding dong, that's your rib bone!" I never felt it before. I thought it was a growth. And then another night I'll feel around and think, "What's this?" So I have a tendency to get a little freaked out about my deflating body.*

Karina had more fears about something being wrong with her body when she was thin than when she was obese. It was going to take some time to learn this body that felt so strange and lumpy to her. Other women even spoke about not knowing how to dress anymore.

PENELOPE: *I don't have to be Mom's good girl anymore. I'm grown up, and I've got a better body. And Mom's not going to tell me how to dress anymore. So what am I going to do? How am I going to dress?*

It is curious how Penelope starts off by sounding rebellious and ends by sounding confused. After years of being told to cover up, to wear muumuus and body-concealing, desexualized clothing, she was fed up. She was ready to break out. Then it occurred to her that she didn't know how to do this—that she hadn't a clue what to wear after a lifetime of considering clothes as blankets under which to hide. Penelope was forty-one years old.

As mentioned earlier, some of the people we interviewed found all of the questions raised by the weight loss complex and disturbing enough to seek professional help in trying to increase their arsenal of coping skills. Some commented on the irony of needing help now that they had lost so much weight, when they had not even thought of it while severely obese.

TED: *Many problems are still there after the weight loss. The weight was so connected to my identity that it was easy to hide behind it. I had never seen a therapist when I was heavy, but I see one now to deal with that.*

Whether or not they were engaged in therapy or attended support groups, almost all of the folks we interviewed commented on how long it took to sort through all the unexpected questions raised by the surgery and weight loss. Years after his procedure, Rex commented, "I'm still trying to figure out which problems were weight-related and which were not." Abby chose a more poetic way of letting us know that it had been a long, hard journey toward the holy grail of self-knowledge when she said, "I have literally walked 250 pounds off. Thousands of miles, you know."

Losing the Pounds and Finding Your Self

The single most powerful benefit of the obesity surgery as recounted by most of our interviewees was the journey toward self-discovery. It was also the least expected of all the benefits and challenges. How could they have known that obesity surgery was going to revolutionize the way they viewed their selves, not just their bodies? It did not seem that predictable, yet, as Karina says, "It's not really about the body. It's more of a cerebral thing." It may seem obvious after the fact, but it was not obvious at all prior to the surgery. The changes that occurred were simply not in the realm of the foreseeable for most people.

RONALD: *The biggest thing out of the surgery . . . you have got to be ready for change. I have always been a person who didn't like change. I liked things to stay the same. But you had better be ready for change with this surgery because every day brings a new challenge.*

URSULA: *I'm not sure emotionally I was ready for the changes that it brought about.*

Many people wished they had been a little more prepared for the revolution ahead. Many wondered if there wasn't some way that prospective patients could receive preoperative training to deal with the challenges they did not even know were coming. They were thankful for the seminar on weight loss and the information about postsurgical diets, but some expressed a need for more in-depth preparation.

ERICA: *There is a major detail missing from the brochures explaining the impact of surgery. We hear a lot about nutritional support, but no one talks about what the weight loss does to your life.*

Maybe there is no way to be completely prepared for that type of impact, but certainly one could benefit from hearing about potential changes and from rehearsing some of the skills that may be a little rusty after many years of obesity.

LAWRENCE: *I think if your frame of mind is right, it's a neat experience, if you have the appropriate skills to deal with it. You know, it's scary, but it's neat. You know, there's a fine line between excitement and fear.*

The magnitude of psychological change reported by most of our interviewees would be challenging for anyone, but it might have been particularly difficult for folks whose self-esteem was very low to begin with. Many of the people we interviewed reported substantial detriments in their self-esteem prior to the surgery. The self-esteem deficits were not just body-esteem deficits, and they didn't all go away after surgery. Decades of severe obesity had made many of them feel very insecure on multiple fronts. That meant that, postsurgery, they would have to face challenges, especially social ones, without the self-assuredness of a healthy, well-established self-concept.

LAWRENCE: *I feel it's very important to be psychologically ready for it. I think it's very important that people are ready for the emotional changes that are going to come. Although . . . I still think there's probably no way to prepare somebody for it. I think you have to have the necessary skills available for it. You have to have good self-esteem. And that's hard in a fat person, because most of us don't.*

Brandon, on the other hand, did not experience the emotional and psychological changes as difficult. His experience of the massive change was more like an epiphany. As far as he was concerned, the surgery itself had just done it. It had been an overnight psychological transformation for him. And considering that he still weighed 435 pounds when we interviewed him eight months after the surgery, it does seem that his psychological change may have occurred at the same time that he made the very decision to have the surgery. Clearly, he was still severely obese.

BRANDON: *My attitude is totally different now than it ever has been. It's really strange to me because it's not something that I had to work at. The psychological changes just occurred as a result of the surgery. And I don't think these changes were attempts to motivate myself, and I don't think they were learned responses. I think that there is something going on either physiologically or psychologically as a direct result of the surgery. Some kind of change.*

The gains in self-discovery, challenging or easy, were experienced by most as overwhelmingly positive. Enhanced feelings of freedom, self-efficacy, and self-worth predominated. Taking responsibility for their lives felt good and solid and real. For some, this new sense of responsibility was a general guideline that now drove their overall search for meaning and happiness.

MAGGIE: *The surgery has helped me come to terms with what I was searching for. I have become stronger in the belief that I have to take responsibility for my own life.*

For others, it was very specific. Now a commitment was a commitment, a promise, a promise. No more excuses.

GORDON: *When you lose the weight, you are going to find out something about yourself. And don't be scared of this because it's a process. "I'm going to have to face my fears, face when I make a promise to my son or make a promise to myself that this is what I want to do and just do it."*

For most people, this assuming of responsibility incurred huge increases in their sense of self-efficacy. They felt open, full of potential, and capable of mastering their universe. What a contrast from life in a recliner!

DAPHNE: *Weight always devastated me. Weight was always on my mind. Now for the first time in my life, I feel free from fat thinking. I have my life back. I have a new perspective. I want to achieve more. I have higher expectations. I'll tear my house down and remodel it myself.*

Tearing her house down and remodeling it herself seemed a great metaphor for the internal personal reconstruction that Daphne and most of our interviewees had engaged in.

KARINA: *I know I have unlimited potential, and I never believed that before. I know I can finish school and do what I need to do. And it will take as long as it takes, just like my weight loss.*

HELENA: *I can be me. I don't need a man in my life to survive. I can stand on my own two feet. I can be self-sufficient. I've got the intelligence. I've got the personality. I've got the self-respect.*

Most of our interviewees had gotten a taste of freedom, and they were hooked. In Brandon's words, "It's a whole new type of life, a whole new type of freedom." It is the liberation of knowing that we have control over our lives—that we get to determine much of it. And that is the major benefit of taking responsibility for our lives. It spurs us to action and makes us go out there and get what we want. It also opens up our minds to possibilities we hadn't even let ourselves imagine prior to the weight loss.

HELENA: *When you lose the weight, your mind becomes so open and so receptive to so many things. Every month I attend a book club, and I would never have done that before because I would have been afraid to share my thoughts.*

We may not always succeed, but we are going to succeed a whole lot more than if we stay in the house and decide that we are doomed by our circumstances. The comfort of that is shallow. Most of our interviewees found themselves and felt nourished by the discovery. As Talia said, "Now I eat a lot less, but I am feeding my spirit." Penelope experienced it as a coming out.

PENELOPE: *I was always behind the scenes. Now I'm a little more willing to say who and what I am.*

Some folks even worried that the pendulum may have swung too far from the extreme of self-abnegation to maybe a little bit of selfishness. Abby's attitude was that if it took some selfishness to recover herself, so be it.

ABBY: *I've worked really hard to get here, and I'm not going to backtrack. If somebody thinks it's selfish, I can't care. We have to be a little selfish. I've had to teach myself that it's okay to fulfill my needs apart from what I provide for my family. I may have to take little something from some areas of my life to fill out others, but I have to do it. If I don't, I'm going to be right back in that chair, 400 pounds and not accomplishing a thing.*

Orianna, on the other hand, felt it might be time to strike a better balance between her old self-effacing self to the new more demanding and maybe slightly self-involved one.

ORIANNA: *I've gotten more wrapped up in myself, and I really need to back off from that, and I'm aware of that. Now when I want something, I want it now and I don't wait. Part of me thinks it's justified because of what I missed out on. I guess I feel I'm owed it. I feel I was cheated for so long. Now I want it with more hunger than I ever wanted food, which blows me away because I always hated the sentiment of "Nothing tastes as good as thin feels."*

It hardly seems surprising that these individuals felt intoxicated with their having found themselves after so many years of feeling lost. One of the challenges ahead of them would be to settle into a sense of self that was healthy but that also considered the needs of others. That would have to be calibrated along with so many other aspects of their new lives.

But adjustments aside, the gain in self-appreciation was experienced as incredibly healing. A lifetime of denigration was fading, and these individuals could start feeling positively about themselves. It is hard to argue with the benefit of that.

> HELENA: *The self-esteem is the center of the wheel, and all the other things in your life are the spokes to help the wheel turn. But if you don't have the self-esteem, then you don't have the spokes.*

For Lawrence and many others, the experience was life changing to an extent they could not have imagined.

> LAWRENCE: *I always thought I was a bad person because I was fat. And to realize you are not a bad person is just overwhelming. It just struck me one day at the doctor's office three to six months after the surgery. That I wasn't bad. And to think I had felt that way for twenty-eight years! It's overwhelming.*

It is quite possible that Lawrence had not been fully aware that he thought he was a bad person until he stopped feeling that way. The sadness he felt for the twenty-eight years of self-depreciation was significant, but it was overshadowed by the relief of having been at last released from that prison. Abby had credited her mother for always having made her feel loved and special even when she was at her highest weight and the target of everyone's derision. Abby felt that this unconditional love and regard had made it possible for her to maintain her self-esteem even when severely obese. It had given her the strength to have the surgery. Drawing from this experience she had some advice for us.

> ABBY: *If you ever have to deal with overweight people in your practice, teach them that they are important, that God loves them, and that no matter what anybody else says or does, that they are loved and they are important.*

Many of our interviewees spoke of their life after the surgery as a rebirth. Many saw themselves as having lived out the fantasy many of us occasionally have of erasing the past and starting again. Maybe erasing the past was not as easy as some had expected, but they definitely got to push the reset button, and it was a source of joy and hope for the vast majority of them.

LAWRENCE: *You know how people say, "Man, if I could just be reborn and do it all over again?" Well, I think literally what I went through was a rebirth. And that's neat. It's neat to go through that, and I feel lucky to have experienced it.*

Part II

Mapping the Journey

CHAPTER 6

Greater Than the Weight of Our Parts

Making Sense of It All

What the surgeon does in the operating room is nothing compared to what the patient has to do every day in the long term.

—FRANCES

Everyone is fascinated by before-and-after photographs, no matter the topic. We are drawn to the results of transformations, from bad to good and from good to bad. The transformation of a city from hamlet to metropolis, from bustling market district to bombed-out remains, from ghetto to gentrified neighborhood. We especially like to see transformations in people from homely to pretty, from old to young, from scarred to smoothed over. How many of us have been channel surfing, caught one of those makeover shows unintentionally, and then felt compelled to suffer through drawn-out story lines and countless commercials just to see the end result? It is irresistible.

Well, our interviewees had their very own before-and-after photos. Some were dramatic, others less so. At the time of the interview, Brandon and Talia had not yet lost that much weight comparatively, as they were only months out of surgery. They had both lost about 90 pounds. The change was more noticeable in Talia, who had started at 355, than it was in Brandon, who had started at 525. Generally speaking, "lightweights" didn't require as much weight loss to look very changed. Three years after the surgery, Natalie had lost 100 pounds, but that had taken her from 225 pounds down to 125, a very big difference. Maggie scored very high on the before-and-after shock meter, as she had lost 350 pounds. Orianna was also up there, with a weight loss of 300 pounds one year after surgery. It was a transformation that made many of them unrecognizable to others and even to themselves.

At first they didn't recognize their own "after" photos, and, eventually, they didn't recognize the "before" ones. These photos were very important to most of the folks we interviewed. They showed them to us, they showed them to other people in their lives, and sometimes they simply just sat with them. The photos served different purposes at different times with different people. Sometimes they were used as medals or trophies. Look at this! Look at what I did! At other times, the before photos were used as reminders of how bad things had been, and some people would cry over them, retroactively giving themselves the sympathy and compassion they had never gotten. The before photos also served as motivators to stay on course with the new lifestyle. Look at that! That's how you'll end up again if you don't watch it. Sometimes, the before photographs were even used as weapons, as when Doris angrily asked the flirtatious gas station attendant if he would have served the woman in the photo.

Curiously, some of our interviewees seemed a little stunned themselves when they showed us the people they were. It was as if even they couldn't believe the change, were it not for the photos. The photos were concrete evidence of the very long journey they had traveled. They had put one foot in front of another, and the incremental progress, dramatic at times and imperceptible at others, had reached a critical mass. We got the impression that were it not for the before-and-after shots, even *they* might have forgotten where they had come from and what they had done to arrive at their destination. The photos certainly didn't show what had happened in between. And as Frances so clearly expressed, it was very important to understand what had happened in between.

FRANCES: *If you think the surgery is magic and that magic made you lose the weight, then it must be really frightening to walk around thinking that your whole life hinges on magic. What if the magic goes away? The man goes away, the job goes away, and your whole life goes away.*

Getting from Before to After

As is the case in all journeys, it is important to map the journey from clinically severe obesity to obesity surgery to sustained weight loss. Ideally, we want to map a journey prior to departure so we don't get lost, so we know what to expect, so we make good time, so we know what's worth stopping for. Of course, it is not possible to predict everything that can happen along the way, but a good part of it is relatively foreseeable. Most of our interviewees were trying to map their journey out of severe obesity after the fact. Although they had received more presurgical preparation than was common at the time, they had still felt quite lost through the whole process, not knowing what to expect at the next turn in the road. They had learned much along the way and could now tell us a lot about the path. Their sharing of their pioneering experiences makes it possible for us and others to try to map this journey. Armed with this knowledge, people considering or undergoing the surgery can do so with as much preparation as possible. So let's take a look at this map.

The journey started with the *contemplation of surgery*. As we heard in our interviews, this decision was not easy. Barriers to taking the leap were:

- fear of the procedure

- fear of complications

- mistrust of doctors

- shame and embarrassment about not having been able to diet successfully

- fear that others would judge surgery as "the easy way out"

- embarrassment about appearing desperate

- fear of not being able to adhere to the postsurgical diet

- denial of the effects of clinically severe obesity

- hopelessness and depression
- resignation and self-defeating tendencies

That is quite a long list of pretty formidable barriers. Yet our interviewees overcame them because they reached a point at which they judged the incentives to simply be greater. The barriers were overcome by an intense desire to:

- stay alive
- be healthy and reduce comorbid diseases
- envision a future
- enjoy life
- feel attractive
- have a successful romantic relationship and maybe get married
- save a marriage
- have a family
- be able to parent and take care of children properly
- model healthy and life-affirming behavior for children
- unburden spouses and family members
- go to work or advance in career or go back to school
- be active and mobile
- have a social life
- rediscover one's personality
- effectively manage and keep one's household

These incentives also gave rise to a set of expectations that were not fulfilled in all cases. That was surprising and disappointing for some interviewees. For others, failed expectations served as an opportunity for self-reflection and growth. Maybe weight loss would facilitate the attainment of these wishes, but weight loss alone would not be enough. They would have to roll up their sleeves and address aspects of their behaviors and personalities that were maybe interfering with the happiness, weight aside.

The first six months after the surgery are often referred to as the *honeymoon period*. These first few months are generally characterized by the most dramatic weight loss. On average, 50 percent of the excess weight will be lost during this time period with what feels like little effort. Our interviewees, much like other patients, recalled experiencing difficulty tolerating many foods and getting the required nutrients. During this period, a great deal of time and energy was spent on healing from the surgery, learning to eat right, and doing what was necessary not to get sick. For some gastric bypass patients, this period is the time when "dumping" is experienced most frequently. Dumping can be caused by eating too much in one setting or consuming foods high in carbohydrates or fat. The consequence is a medley of uncomfortable symptoms such as nausea, dizziness, sweats, vomiting, or diarrhea. The experience is so unpleasant that in essence it worked as a type of aversion therapy to condition against eating the wrong things or too much or too fast.[1] Not every gastric bypass patient experiences dumping, and for those who do initially, their low tolerance to these nutrients is likely to dissipate. It is thus unwise to rely on dumping as a way to change your behavior. Dumping, however, resulted in some patients being able to avoid foods they used to crave prior to the surgery. Some were shocked to report that they even "forgot" to eat sometimes, an unheard-of occurrence prior to the surgery.

We did not interview anybody who had been out of surgery less than six months, but they recalled being amazed and giddy at the sight of their shrinking bodies during those early months. What had been the most difficult thing in the world to them, losing weight, now seemed ridiculously easy. Reinforcement was at its height during this period. Every time they stepped on the scale, the number would be closer to their goal. The mirror reinforced them each time they looked in it and saw a smaller reflection of themselves. The people in their lives were also stunned at the change and told them repeatedly how well they were doing and how much better they looked. That was a lot of stroking. It was also a time of big emotion that they could no longer soothe with their old habits. It was very shocking to change so dramatically, and, as we have read in the previous chapters, not all of the emotion experienced early on was exhilarating. There was also regret for not having had the surgery sooner and embarrassment for having done it at all, not to mention a great deal of confusion. Except now, sitting down with a tub of Häagen-Dazs was no longer an option, not even the bad option it had always been. It would more than likely make them ill, and it certainly wasn't recommended. And so another challenge at this stage was to grieve for food and the role it had played in their lives. For some, it was like saying good-bye to an old friend—an old friend that had gotten them in a world of pain and trouble, but an old friend nonetheless.

Despite these challenges, motivation and optimism were at their highest during the honeymoon period because changes were rapid and the external reinforcement was everywhere and frequent. This makes the honeymoon period a crucial one for obesity surgery patients. If healthy habits can be in-stated and well established during this time of high optimism and reinforce-ment, it is more likely that these habits will be adopted for the long term, when they will be needed even more.

The third identifiable part of the surgery journey out of severe obesity is the six-to-twelve-month period we call the *settling-in period*. During this period, the weight loss slows down substantially. Those dramatic losses evi-dent from week to week that were so thrilling are starting to disappoint. The weight loss continues but at a much slower pace. Typically, weight loss is at 50 to 80 percent of excess weight by the end of the first year. This slowing down of the weight loss pace can be very scary and even disheartening to patients. They had gotten used to the quick pace, to the exhilaration of it. As scary as losing weight very quickly was at times, for some, the settling-in pe-riod was scarier. What if the weight loss stops? What if I gain?

The slowing down of the weight loss was also accompanied by the abil-ity to tolerate a greater range and quantity of foods. Although it was pleas-ant to not feel as restricted as in those first few months and to lose the fear of getting violently ill in public, this was also a dangerous development. It meant that they could eat more of what wasn't good for them. For many of our interviewees, previously craved foods that had lost their appeal during the honeymoon period had started to look appetizing again. Some, such as

Maggie, openly reported that they tested the limits of what they could tolerate by trying desserts, as well as fried and fast foods. In the honeymoon period cheating was almost impossible, but in the settling-in period it was possible. This was the first time since the surgery that willpower had to start kicking in. Now there were choices, and with them came responsibility.

The settling-in period was also characterized by a slow decrease in the amount of external reinforcement coming our interviewees' way. People had gotten used to their weight loss, and the weekly changes were also nowhere near as impressive. Whereas in the honeymoon period that external reinforcement had propped up some of our interviewees, in the settling-in period they had to rely much more heavily on their own intrinsic motivation and reinforcement. It was also during this period that our interviewees experienced most of their gains in self-esteem, confidence, and assertiveness. These essentially positive developments had also shaken up their jobs and relationships, resulting in some tumult.

Most of our interviewees were in the settling-in period, and their experiences seemed varied to some extent. At six months, Talia still felt like she was in the honeymoon period.

> TALIA: *My birthday is six months from now, and I am planning to weigh 200 pounds by then. All I have to do is lose 10 pounds a month. When I hit 200 I'm going to have the biggest party! The biggest pool party! And I'm going invite everybody. We're going to celebrate my 200-pound body!*

At eight months, Brandon also still sounded like he was in the honeymoon period. He was very far from his goal weight, but was full of optimism and confident he would get there. Jessica and Karina, also eight months out, had both lost approximately 200 pounds and showed no signs of a weakening commitment. Neither did Orianna, who had lost close to 300 pounds in one year. Erica, on the other hand, had stopped losing weight after seven or so months and was starting to feel discouraged by that and by the fact that many of her expectations about how the weight loss would change her life had not yet come to pass.

The fourth part of the journey out of obesity was the twelve-to-eighteen-month period we call the *Are we there yet? period*. The honeymoon was definitely over at this point. Weight loss was accomplished through painstaking daily commitment and changes in lifestyle and other behaviors. The surgery could no longer be relied upon for weight loss. To further complicate matters, most foods could now be tolerated in more or less normal quantities. The danger was that old habits could start to make a full-fledged return, and some folks became less vigilant of the lifestyle changes that needed to be maintained.

The Are we there yet? period was also characterized by a near cessation of external reinforcement. People who knew our interviewees prior to the surgery had gotten used to the thinner versions of them, and new acquaintances did not know they had been severely obese to begin with. So the compliments and kudos pretty much stopped coming. In addition, most of our interviewees expressed frustration with the fact that their own mental image of themselves, their self-concept, had not caught up with the weight loss. They complained that they still felt like fat people and were afraid that the old feelings of insecurity might never completely go away. By the time folks got to the Are we there yet? period, most of the major life changes that had been expected to occur as a consequence of weight loss had either started to happen, already happened, or were not going to happen at all. This made it more difficult to maintain the motivation still necessary to maintain weight loss. Either folks had gotten what they wanted and thus felt a decrease in drive, or they were so disappointed that the dieting and lifestyle changes hardly seemed worth it. Virtually all of our interviewees in the Are we there yet? period still seemed motivated, but that may be due to a bias in our sample. The obesity surgery patients who agreed to be interviewed by us may have been the particularly motivated ones. What often happens in obesity surgery clinics is that patients stop returning, and they are lost to follow-up. One can probably surmise that a good number of them ended up having less-than-good outcomes.

Eighteen months and beyond, the *deciding-to-stay period* is the last leg of the journey out of clinically severe obesity. Usually, weight loss has completely ceased by this point. In a significant number of surgery patients, there is even some weight gain. The physiological effects of the surgery are no longer actively working toward weight loss, and only the individual can stop him- or herself from making poor choices about eating, activities, and lifestyle. If the person has achieved his or her goal weight, the trick now is to stay there. Fear of regaining weight is common at this stage, although fear alone does not appear to be enough of a deterrent.

It is also at this point in the journey that the heaviest individuals presurgically started complaining about sagging skin and started investigating interventions to correct this problem. As we saw in our group, this period was also characterized by some disappointment that problems previously blamed on weight had not been resolved. In many of our interviewees, the deciding-to-stay period was also the period in which they accomplished a great deal of personal growth. They went back and confronted the psychological, behavioral, and relational issues that had contributed to their obesity. They looked closely at themselves and tried to address those aspects of their characters that were keeping them from fulfillment. A number of our interviewees in the deciding-to-stay period were 10 to 15 pounds heavier than their target weight. They would lose these 10 to 15 pounds and then regain them. As long as those pounds did not continue to rise, it was a dance many of them had become accustomed to, although the terror of returning to obesity would remain in the background. The following outline shows visually the five stages of the journey.

The Journey Out of Obesity

Departure Point: Contemplating Obesity Surgery

Reasons Not to Go	Reasons to Go
Danger in surgery	Health
Shame and embarrassment	Emotional well-being
Judgment of others	Improved relationships
Return to dieting	Better parenting
Obesity not that bad	Work and career opportunities
Nothing will work	Increased attractiveness

Zero to Six Months: The Honeymoon Period
Physiologically Driven Dramatic Weight Loss

Pit Stops	Lookouts
Healing from surgery	Huge reinforcement
Learning to eat right—getting right nutrients	Attractiveness
Avoiding dumping—foods that aren't tolerated	Optimism
Some regret, embarrassment, grieving of food	Motivation
	Gains in self-esteem and assertiveness
	Health improvements

Six to Twelve Months: The Settling-In Period
Weight Loss Slows Down

Pit Stops	Lookouts
Being careful about higher tolerance for foods	Pleasant decrease in restriction
Getting return of cravings under control	Pleasant decrease in bouts of dumping
Responsibility for choices	Readjustments at work and in relationships
Panic about slowdown of weight loss	
Resisting the urge to test food limits	

Twelve to Eighteen Months: The Are We There Yet? Period
Weight loss proceeds only through commitment to eating and lifestyle change

Pit Stops	Lookouts
Watch for decrease in motivation	Full extent of gains in life changes really evident
Watch for the return of old habits	Improvements in relationships, parenting, career
Need to rely on intrinsic reinforcement;	Start to see yourself in a different light
compliments on weight loss start winding down	Self-reflection and self-evaluation
Mental image lagging behind weight loss	

Eighteen Months and Beyond: The Deciding-to-Stay Period
Weight loss has stopped—maybe some regain

Pit Stops	Lookouts
Remain vigilant about maintenance	Explore reasons for obesity
Make good choices	Self-improvement and personal growth

Born Again?

And so our interviewees generously shared with us stories about their journeys that helped us draw up a map of what others might expect. But the idea of a journey or a map to chart that journey was our metaphor, not theirs. When we asked them what it had felt like to go back to their lives after leaving the operating room, many of them used an altogether different metaphor. The core process that emerged from our interviewees' description of life after obesity surgery was the metaphor of a rebirth. As demonstrated by the before-and-after pictures, the surgery seemed to be a landmark in their psychic landscape that created a clear, dichotomous division between their old presurgical life and their new postsurgical one. Interviewees presented this concept of transformation and rebirth in various forms, such as getting a second chance at life, becoming visible to a world in which they had once felt insignificant, or developing a newfound sense of freedom from the preoperative entrapment in their own bodies. Interviewees who recalled severe preoperative psychosocial impairment and desperation tended to experience the most dramatic rebirth and transformation process. Similarly, interviewees who were massively obese typically lost weight more rapidly than the average patient, perhaps making this evolution more remarkable.

> LAWRENCE: *You know how people always say, "Man, if I could just be reborn and do it all over again"? Well, what we go through is literally a rebirth. And that's neat. It's neat to go through that. I feel lucky to have experienced it.*

Although interviewees who had suffered from extreme preoperative weight-related physical and psychosocial impairment were likely to experience this transformation with the greatest intensity, numerous patients who began this process as lightweights also described a similar phenomenon. The experience of surgery as rebirth and transformation set up a dividing line between the old presurgical self and the new postsurgical self. Every aspect of life after surgery seemed to be compared to its presurgical analog in the search for contrasts. Confirming that life had indeed changed was important, not just to justify the physical trauma and expense of the surgery but also to keep one motivated for the ongoing dietary struggle.

Tension in Change

The essential changes that people experienced shortly after the surgery consisted primarily of:

- improvements in physical health
- the ability to move around and be active
- the lifting of severe depression and anxiety
- greater physical attractiveness as perceived by self and others
- the ability to envision a future with potential

These changes seemed pretty universal, and all were positive, at face value. Most of our interviewees had gone from constricted lives of immobility and limited life choices to lives with expanding horizons. Possibility was suddenly all around them. Hard not to cheer for that! However, change almost always generates tension, and, as we read in the preceding chapters, these very positive changes triggered a cascade of other unexpected developments that posed some formidable challenges for many of the patients. Most of these challenges could broadly be organized into the categories of self, relationship, and skill deficits.

In terms of self, we saw our interviewees struggle with:

- *Feelings of vulnerability.* As the weight disappeared, they were left without its familiar "protection." They now had to face the real reasons they failed or succeeded.

- *Confusion about cause and effect.* It was at times difficult to realize that the weight could be blamed for only so much—that maybe something in their personalities or skill sets was the accurate causal attribution for a particular failure. They also couldn't make more of their successes than what they were. They could no longer magnify their gains by saying, "And I got the job, despite being this heavy!"

- *Not knowing how much to focus on themselves.* After a lifetime in the practice of self-effacement, some now wondered how much self-focus was appropriate or enough or too much. Were they being selfish in demanding certain gratifications, or was it okay to do so?

- *Changes in values and life goals.* These changed dramatically for some folks as they rewrote their life scripts and reshuffled priorities.

- *Reflections on the role of obesity in their lives.* Some mourned the years lost in the fog of obesity and self-defeatism and wondered why they had given up their power so easily. Most were aghast when the weight loss showed them the huge role that obesity had played in their lives and relationships.

Relationships also presented significant challenges:

- *Friendships were changed.* As roles shifted, some friendships became stronger, and others just didn't make it. The experience left some people with an increased awareness of how great their friends actually were. Lost friendships were met with resignation, sadness, anger, and relief.

- *Marriages and romantic relationships were destabilized.* Outcomes of this destabilization ranged from great improvement to dissolution, probably contingent on the quality of the relationship presurgically. Those marriages in which the obesity played a significant role in the stability of the relationship couldn't take the hit. A couple of women opted for the surgery as a first step in liberating themselves from dysfunctional unions, whereas others were completely blindsided by the effects of the weight loss on these relationships. In our interviews, we saw a lot of distress regarding the impact of the surgery on marriages, as patients struggled with jealousy, insecurity, and hostility.

- *Families of origin were impacted.* Although they appeared more resilient than nonkin relationships, we got the impression that in the long term, these systems were also reconfigured. The thing with families of origin is that, even when things aren't comfortable, most people don't file for "divorce" from their parents or siblings. Most of us endure the difficulties. They are who they are. But they are where we came from. And that's hard to leave.

⊚ *Conflict and anger about newfound attention.* This was one of the more surprising findings in our study. The women we spoke to felt especially offended by the contrast in their treatment by others pre- and post-surgery. It was hard for many of them to simply revel in the new compliments and come-ons knowing that just months earlier they had been the targets of these new suitors' open derision.

Finally, our interviewees had to deal with multiple "how-to" problems. There were so many experiences from which a lifetime of obesity had shielded them that they literally did not have the skills that other people take for granted:

⊚ *Responding to kindness.* Many of our interviewee reported that they never learned how to accept a compliment—sadly, because they recalled having been given so few. Even the compliments they had fielded were met with skepticism. Was it a joke? Was there an ulterior motive for the sweet nothings? Now they found themselves having to respond to a barrage of compliments.

⊚ *Navigating the dating scene.* Dating felt strange and even dangerous. Some didn't know how to act and or what the "rules" were. When was it okay to have sex, and was it okay just to say, "No, I don't want to"?

⊚ *Standing up for self.* As they became more assertive, several of our interviewees struggled to find the appropriate balance between stating their needs and being too demanding. Where was the line between an appropriate demand for their rights or something they felt they deserved and being aggressive, pushy, and entitled?

⊚ *Making lifestyle and dietary changes.* They all had to learn to eat in a completely different way.

⊚ *Using food to cope with emotions.* Our interviewees had to learn how to cope with negative emotions without turning to food for comfort. This meant the development of a whole new set of skills for dealing with frustration or sadness or anger.

We did not interview a single person who regretted having this surgery, but we did interview a lot of people who found the whole experience to be quite challenging. There is no question that the changes experienced by most of them would easily be classified as essentially positive in nature. But that does not mean that things simply got better for them right away. Many had to work very hard to ensure that the challenges posed by these changes resulted in growth rather than in withdrawal and defeatism.

DAPHNE: *Right after the surgery, there is this part of you that thinks, "I'm cured. I'm automatically going to lose weight." But the surgery alone only works by itself for the first several months, maybe a year. But then you have to take over. You have to establish your new habits and your new patterns, and that can be rough because you are confronting a lot of issues that you never confronted before.*

What Is Success?

Obesity surgery is an incredibly effective tool for losing massive amounts of weight, but it does not come with a handbook to negotiate successfully the challenges that one might face when that weight comes off. Everyone in our study experienced some form of tension out of the changes that occurred postsurgically. These tensions existed in different areas and to varying degrees. We believe the successful negotiation of that tension may be the single most important determinant of surgery-outcome success. But first, let's investigate what we mean by a successful surgery outcome.

We could define it simply by number of pounds lost. Alternately, we could shift the emphasis over to quality of life. These may be closely related for most people, but maybe not as closely related as one might think. Most patients come out of surgery with a target weight as per their doctor. The first few months are relatively easy, and the weight comes off almost miraculously. Yes, there is a dietary regimen, but the speed with which it all works at the beginning is astounding to most people undergoing it. After a few months, as we saw, the weight loss slows down. This slowing down usually coincides with patients starting to feel temptations for foods that are off the acceptable list and a general tendency to try to experiment to see what they can get away with. What if someone decides that, although they are not at the doctor-recommended target weight, they have made the quality-of-life gains they wished for and that this is good enough for them? It could be that they have lost enough weight to resolve their serious medical conditions, increase their activity level, and have higher self-esteem, yet they remain substantially overweight. They may determine their weight loss is sufficient and that there is no urgent need for further efforts.

> REX: *I set my own weight loss goal that within a year and a half I would lose 100 pounds. I say to myself that is good enough, but when is enough, enough? I keep saying to myself that I'm happy where I'm at, but a little voice in my head tells me, "You said the same thing when you were 300 pounds."*

Was it a reasonable decision for a couple of our interviewees to stop losing when they felt happy enough? Or could it be that they were just engaging in the kind of denial that kept them obese in the first place? It's hard to know, but it seems reasonable to us to bank on the quality-of-life measure of surgery success. After all, what is the point of losing weight if it isn't to improve one's life? Continuing to feel miserable and unhappy after weight loss could hardly be considered a good outcome.

Now it happens to be that at approximately twenty-four months after surgery many patients start to gain weight. We have all noticed that certain celebrities whom we saw a few months after obesity surgery look quite a bit heavier a couple of years out, although normally not quite at presurgical levels. After more than thirty years of research in the field of obesity surgery, we still are not entirely sure why this regain occurs.[2] We know that it has to do with developing maladaptive eating habits, such as skipping meals and then overeating, or carelessly snacking throughout the day. But why would patients engage in maladaptive eating behaviors after undergoing such an invasive procedure with all the attendant costs and risks? The simple answer is that doing things that feel good are simply hard to drop. And eating feels good. The postsurgical regimen can be tough, and some people revert back to old, familiar, and comforting patterns. So what differentiates those who do return to maladaptive eating from those who do not? We think the answer might be a little more complex than "Eating feels good, so I'm going to do it." We are suggesting that it has to do with quality of life. If your quality of life improves, then the effort is worth it. If your quality of life does not improve or if it gets even worse, what would be the motivation for putting in the effort to lose weight or maintain the weight lost? A study of twenty gastric bypass patients found that fear of confrontation and difficulty coping with life's demands were characteristic of patients who lost the least amount of weight.[3]

This leads us to the conclusion that the success with which patients negotiate the tension-generating changes effected by obesity surgery and its consequent weight loss may be an important determinant of surgery outcome, and maybe the most important one. There is little question that dramatic weight loss poses a challenge. Knowing how to deal with it may be more crucial than the surgeon's incision or stapling or Lap-Band insertion in ensuring that weight stays off. We have developed a model that illustrates how we think this process might work. The onus in this model is on the patient's ability to cope with the tension generated by the changes. To briefly recap the model of the postobesity surgery process, as illustrated below, the surgery is experienced by many patients as a type of transformation or rebirth. The transformation creates a dichotomy between one's presurgical and postsurgical lives. The contrast between these "two lives" is characterized by some essential and fairly universal changes that are mostly positive in nature, such as improvements in physical and mental health. For some people, however, these changes have a wide impact on their lives in ways that create a certain level of destabilization and tension. The tension does not necessarily mean that outcomes are negative; rather, even essentially positive changes can produce a number of challenges in the areas of self-concept, relationships, and the acquisition of skills. Coping and adapting to these changes are significant parts of the recovery process. The extent to which folks are able to efficaciously negotiate or navigate these challenges to arrive at a new, more satisfying, and functional stability will have an impact on the motivation to continue adhering to the weight loss regimen once the "magic" of the surgery has been depleted. In other words, the ability of patients to cope with the changes and improve the quality of their lives may determine the long-term success of the surgery in ensuring both an optimal weight and an improved quality of life. Of course, this model needs to be tested in scientific studies, but until the data come in, there seems little danger in investing in a systematic attempt to improve the quality of life of postobesity surgery patients. We believe the benefits could be very significant.

Model of the Post–Obesity Surgery Process

Rebirth and Transformation

↓

Creation of Dichotomy Between Presurgery (Old) and Postsurgery (New) Life

|

Essential Changes

Physical health

Mobility

Mental health

Appearance

Assessment of potential

|

Potential Tension Areas

Self-Concept	Social Relations	Skills Acquisition
Vulnerability	Friendship roles	Eating behavior
Causal attributions	Marital/romantic dynamics	Coping with emotions
Self-focus	Family roles	Social skills
Values	Conflict about new attention	Assertiveness
Role of weight in self-concept	Anger about past discrimination	—

|

Negotiation of Tension in Affected Areas

↓

Long-Term Surgery Outcome

CHAPTER 7 **Through Thick and Thin**

Planning for Success

If you are not prepared to start fighting some of the
fights that happen when you lose the shield of fat,
you are going to backslide and have problems.
—FRANCES

When individuals opt for obesity surgery, they make a big investment. They
have to take time off work, they cannot fulfill family duties for a while, they
risk surgical complications, they spend money. Ensuring that this investment will result in good returns is a priority. For most people, that means
selecting a good surgeon, getting in physical shape for the surgery (including
losing some weight beforehand), and, of course, following the recommended
postsurgical diet, exercise, and medication regimen. We think preparing for
some of the potential emotional and relational consequences of the surgery
might be almost as important as dieting and drugs. We also think that this
preoperative preparation can be followed up in the weeks and months after
the surgery to guide folks through some of the challenges as they happen.
Anticipation is important, but getting help when the rubber meets the road
can also be very helpful.

So what might this preparation look like? Based on our research, clinical work, and interviews with many obesity surgery patients, we have developed a program. This program aims to guide patients and their counselors
through the presurgical preparation and postsurgical process with a specific focus on self-concept, relationships, and skill building, as defined by the

"Model of the Post–Obesity Surgery" process we outlined in Chapter 6. We call this program Through Thick and Thin (TTAT) in recognition of the fact that even positive developments can be challenging. It consists of a series of steps that can be implemented with the help of a counselor, in the context of a support group, or on an individual basis by following the guide here suggested. Most people we have spoken to claim that counselors and therapists or counselor-guided support groups were tremendously helpful to them in adapting to the changes that followed surgery and weight loss. Most obesity surgery clinics provide these services or give referrals to professionals who do. Although one could do this work individually, it's harder to do it alone. Most people benefit greatly from peer support and from the guidance of health professionals with experience in this area. The Through Thick and Thin program can thus be used by counselors and support groups to guide their activities and discussions. Although we strongly recommend that individuals considering or undergoing obesity surgery avail themselves of these professional services, we also understand that everybody is different and that access to these services is not universal. Some people favor the solitary approach to working on their issues, whereas others prefer a professionally guided or group-driven effort. For others, these services may not be readily available or affordable. That is why we have tried to design the Through Thick and Thin program so that it can also be followed by individuals, on their own. The point is to be proactive and to reduce the element of surprise in the process of losing weight so that one does not get thrown off-course.

The TTAT program consists of a series of steps and exercises to help you prepare for the changes to come and to help you cope with them once they start to happen. The Presurgical Module consists primarily of education, identification of issues, and discussion of concerns with significant others. The Postsurgical Module consists primarily of the emotional processing of changes and of skills building. Although the steps are here necessarily outlined in a sequential (one step leads to another) fashion, many of them can be worked on at the same time. Some folks will feel they need to spend more time on some steps than others, but the point is to at least consider each one of them, either briefly or at length.

Many people don't realize they need to do this type of work until they have already had the operation. In that case, the entire TTAT program can be followed postsurgically. Although we consider it optimal to go into the surgery with some preparation for the issues that may arise, this does not always happen in the desired order. Some people think they don't need to process anything until they get hit with the after-the-fact reality. Our interviewees showed us that. And that's okay, too. Working through all of these issues after the surgery, instead of before, remains preferable to not reflecting on them at all. It is human nature to not deal with issues until we have to. The really important thing is to deal with them at some point. Timing may be a factor in the obesity surgery process, but, unlike in comedy, timing isn't everything. An outline of the TTAT program is provided below, and a more in-depth elaboration of each step follows:

Through Thick and Thin Program Treatment Steps

Presurgical Module

1 Psychoeducation

2 Identifying and assessing expectations

3 Investigating factors contributing to obesity

4 Investigating the role of weight

5 Identifying instability risk areas

6 Discussing concerns with significant others

7 Brainstorming alternate ways of coping with emotions

8 Formalizing current self-concept

Postsurgical Module

9 Processing the expectation-reality alignment

10 Implementing alternate coping strategies

11 Reconfiguring self-concept

12 Practicing social skills and appropriate assertiveness

13 Communicating with significant others

14 Making plans to live out dreams

Presurgical Module

Step 1. Psychoeducation

Surgical Options. Read everything you can about the different types of surgery available. Investigate how each one works physiologically. Most bariatric clinics will have a Web site outlining the procedures that they offer or brochures they can provide to you. Below are some questions we recommend you explore:

What exactly is done to the stomach?

Do different types of surgeries work best for different people?

What are the potential complications of each procedure, and how common are they?

How are digestion and metabolism changed or affected?

What kind of changes can you expect in your body, hair, skin (both transient and permanent)?

If you have already been in touch with a specific clinic, you may want to ask if you can speak to patients who had the surgery that you are considering. Try to attend a support group. Some clinics have buddy systems, whereby new candidates for the surgery are paired with veterans who can provide information and help them through the process. A selection of resources is available in the "Selected Resources for Public and Health Professionals" section at the end of this book.

The Reconstructive Surgeries. Although most people don't think about sagging skin or reconstructive surgery when they are considering obesity surgery, it is a good idea to get educated about both obesity and reconstructive surgeries simultaneously. Taking into account your preoperative weight and age, you may want to ask a doctor or independently research the following questions:

How much sagging skin and in what areas should you expect it, given your preoperative weight and your target weight?

What are the reconstructive surgeries that might be indicated for you, if you attain your target weight after obesity surgery?

How are these surgeries performed?

What are the associated complications?

What is the cosmetic result you can expect?

What is the recommended time frame for reconstructive surgeries in reference to when the obesity surgery occurred?

Costs and Insurance Coverage. Depending on your preoperative weight and the existence of comorbid diseases, your health insurance company or health management organization may or may not cover costs for the surgery. Usually, this determination is based on the necessity of the operation to your health status. Make sure that you thoroughly investigate whether you will be covered and to what extent. Although many people have their obesity surgery covered, that is not always the case for the reconstructive surgeries. Inquire about your eligibility and get some estimates on the costs of these secondary surgeries. They may not seem that important to you right now, but that might change dramatically with time. Better to be informed at the outset.

The Postsurgical Diet. Remember that even if you have this surgery, dieting will likely remain a constant in your life. The diet that follows most obesity surgeries is relatively specific and restrictive. Know what you are getting into. Research the following questions:

How much should you be eating, how often, and what kinds of food?

How hard or easy do people find it to adhere to the diet?

How long will you remain on liquids or pureed foods?

Will your diet change with time? How?

Are there foods that you can never have?

What kinds of vitamins or medications are necessary after surgery? Why?

Is nutrient insufficiency manageable, and, if not, what will the effects of temporary deficiencies be?

How will the diet affect your ability to go out and dine with friends or colleagues?

Postsurgical Emotional Reactions. Very few people considering obesity surgery wonder how it will affect their mental and emotional well-being. Most fall into the trap of thinking this is simply a weight loss intervention. That is why we wrote this book—because thirty-three people told us how the emotional part was the most challenging and how no one had adequately prepared them for it. Reading this book is a good start. Learning how this surgery has emotionally affected people in the past can only help. Although we all have, in part, a unique set of circumstances, we also share much with others. We can all learn from each other's experiences. In addition to reading this book, you can also do your own research by going online or joining obesity surgery chat rooms.

Be aware of your reaction to the things you read and hear regarding the physical and psychological impact of the surgery and weight loss. Think about how you might feel about and react to the changes. That is why we call this psychoeducation and not just education. It is education about a topic in the context of how you personally will experience it. Accessing information is easier today than it ever has been. There are a number of books that outline what these changes are, and there are, of course, many sites on the Internet that will answer just about any question you may have. We have provided you with a selection of them at the end of this book. There are many others. As you browse, be aware that there are reputable sites and sites that are either trying to sell you something or are high on emotion and low on perspective. Try not to get overly affected by one person's idiosyncratic reaction to the whole procedure. A good surgeon should also make solid educational resources easily available to you so that you end up making your decision with as much information as possible.

Step 2. Identifying and Assessing Expectations

Because happiness depends so much on the alignment of expectations with what can realistically be achieved, it is very important that you identify your expectations about life after weight loss. Be honest with yourself. Even if your expectations are big, admit it. If you think you're going to be a rock star, say so. Better to get the expectations out in the open than to have them disappoint you behind the scenes. Once you have owned them, try to assess how realistic they are and the extent to which you can find evidence for the contention that weight was the barrier to achieving these expectations prior to surgery. Some of the following questions may be helpful in your investigation:

- What do you expect to happen in your life as a consequence of the surgery? It will be easy to answer this question with health-related answers, but try to look deeper inside yourself and identify other expectations that you may secretly harbor. Find true love? A great career? Happiness? It is not stupid to wish any of these things for yourself, but it is crucial to know that you are doing so. It is important, because if you don't acknowledge the true nature of your wishes, a number of things can go amiss:

  you will not be able to assess whether they are realistic

  you will fail to engage in behaviors that might facilitate their attainment

  you might be surprised by feelings of disappointment that you then inaccurately blame on other factors

- How does the weight keep you from achieving these objectives now?

- What reasons other than weight can you think of that are keeping you from achieving these objectives?

Assessing whether your expectations are realistic is difficult, and dreaming big is no sin. It has made people achieve great things. On the other hand, those big dreams don't happen just because we dream them. They require action on our part. Remember that people who are not obese do not have perfect lives either. True love, a great career, and happiness are difficult for everyone to find, regardless of weight. It may be true that these things are even harder to attain under the shadow of extreme obesity, but that doesn't mean that weight loss will clear all obstacles to them. On its own, the surgery is unlikely to be the only tool you need to fulfill expectations. You will have to dig in there and work hard. That's what most of our interviewees told us. Finally, some degree of disappointment is almost inevitable in any life endeavor, and it is likely that you will experience it in regard to what you expected to happen post–weight loss. However, this disappointment can be manageable when you accurately identify its source, accept that it is bound to happen in some measure, and then own the part that is yours to own. At the very least, you can work on the parts you control. Otherwise, you risk bitterness and the development of a mind-set in which you blame the world for your problems. This is an emotional and self-actualization dead-end you don't want to be stuck in.

Step 3. Investigating Factors Contributing to Obesity

We know too much about the biology of clinically severe obesity to attribute all the weight to psychological and social factors. We also know that having a biological predisposition toward obesity does not always result in being overweight. Thus, it seems reasonable in most cases to investigate individual psychological and environmental factors that may have contributed to your obesity. The reason this exercise is important is that it may hold a bunch of clues as to how you can avoid falling back into obesity after the surgery does its "magic." For example:

- Can you identify any experiences or influences in your life that worked to develop or maintain your obesity?
- Are these influences still active in your life?
- What purpose did the obesity serve?
- Was it successful?

Some folks describe themselves as having addictive personalities and believe the answer to why they became obese is in their inability to resist food and the high it gives them. Others talk about a tendency to get depressed or stressed out and about how they used food to quell these negative emotions. Some look to social anxiety as a basis of overeating—rather than face the fear of interactions with others, they simply stayed home and ate on Saturday nights. Yet others speak of environmental influences such as sexual abuse or trauma that they felt led them to desexualize themselves by gaining weight and exiting the arena of sexual interaction. Whatever these reasons may be, we think it is important to identify them because the surgery is not going to excise those reasons. If those reasons are still there after the surgery, you are still going to have to address them. After the surgery, you will probably still have addictive tendencies or social anxiety or an aversion to sexual interactions. These issues are going to need your attention over and above whatever happens as a consequence of the surgery. If these issues are not addressed independently of the weight loss, they might lead you right back into a maladaptive pattern of eating and a return of the obesity that had protected you from them.

Step 4. Investigating the Role of Weight

Highly related to Step 3 is the investigation of the role that weight had come to play in your life. Many of our interviewees were surprised it had had any role at all, other than to make them miserable. However, the vulnerability many of them felt after losing the weight made them realize that the weight had been a major player in their lives, in ways they fully realized only when it was gone. Investigating the role of weight in your life is crucial simply because you are about to lose it. You thus better find out what it was doing. The weight loss will leave some of your needs unmet. Unless you find other ways to deal with whatever the weight was either giving you or protecting you from, you might find yourself yearning to get it back, maybe even subconsciously.

⊙ What are the benefits of being severely obese? This is a difficult question because you might be very defensive about the answer. You might think it is a crazy question. You might even feel slightly offended by it. What could possibly be good about being that obese? But think hard about it. Our interviewees indicated that the weight may have been giving them good excuses not to engage in activities they fear, such as dating or moving up the occupational ladder or fulfilling dreams they doubted they were up to, even without the weight. It may also be giving you an esteem-saving fall-back position for failures. You can blame things on the weight and not on any essential quality in your personality or nature. It is hard to judge the role of weight in your life when you still have it, but we think it's worth an effort in preparation for what is to come.

⊙ What might the weight be protecting you from? If you can, at least, venture to guess what it is protecting you from, then you can start working on your fears, facing your limitations, and striving to be the best that you can be.

⊙ Can you think of any consequences to weight loss that frighten you? Imagine not being overweight and then imagine doing some of the things the weight had stopped you from doing. Imagine having new opportunities in love and work. Would these opportunities possibly threaten certain aspects of your life as they are now?

Identifying the role weight plays in your life may be tantamount to identifying the areas fertile for personal growth. It can be scary to investigate these questions, but, as our interviewees told us, it is also exciting because it means that you are shifting from an attachment to limitations to an attachment to potential. The former feels safer because it is static. The latter holds the promise of more. Whether that promise is fulfilled or not is partly up to you and partly up to life circumstances that necessarily restrict your choices. Some things you can control, and others you can't. It is crucial that you acknowledge and own the ones you have some mastery over to bring success within your reach.

Step 5. Identifying Instability Risk Areas

Although we can all be pretty good at fooling ourselves sufficiently to proceed about our business while the truth exists behind our backs, most of us have some sense of the trouble areas in our lives. Confronting these full-on is hard, but it is usually productive if we are solution oriented. This may be a particularly difficult exercise, but we promise it is also a particularly useful one.

- What aspects of yourself do you feel insecure about?
- How much do you think weight has to do with these insecurities?
- How do you think weight loss will impact these insecurities?
- When you imagine yourself considerably thinner, are these insecurities gone, reduced, or unchanged?

Then there is the whole occupational arena.

- What do you think will happen at work when you lose the weight?
- Will you continue to be satisfied with the job you have, or will you want something better or maybe just different?
- How will your boss or coworkers react if you start expressing your points of view more often or demand equal consideration?

Friendship might also be useful to think about.

- Are your friendships solid, reciprocal relationships in which you get as much as you give?
- If not, what might happen when you start expecting a higher level of reciprocity (give-and-take)?
- Are you prepared to lose some of your less reciprocal friendships?
- What is your role in each of your friendships?
- Is there any chance that some of your friends will feel threatened by your weight loss? How will you deal with that?

As we witnessed in our interviews, marriage and romantic relationships were particularly vulnerable to the destabilizing effect of dramatic weight loss. These may be the relationships most important to consider as you contemplate surgery.

- Are you in this relationship because you value it highly or because you think you can't do any better, given your current weight? If the latter is true, what will happen when you feel you have more options?

- Even if you do value your relationship highly, what might be the reaction of your partner when you start losing the weight and become more attractive, garnering the attention of others? Might there be a possibility of insecurity or jealousy on his or her part?

- How might you allay those fears while protecting your autonomy, if in fact the fears are unfounded?

- What could happen to your feelings and attraction for your partner when you start getting attention from other men or women?

- How do you expect to change in regards to your sexual life?

By considering these questions, you are preparing and thinking ahead about how you might proactively deal with the areas that are mostly likely to be shaken up by the weight loss. Sometimes, simply identifying potential problem areas ensures they never become problems because we are subtly ensuring from the get-go that they don't turn out that way. Yet even if that is not the case, identifying the instability risk areas allows us to confront them and plan ahead. This does not guarantee success, but it makes it much more likely.

Step 6. Discussing Concerns With Significant Others

It is not enough to ask oneself all of these important questions, especially when it comes to maintaining relationships. It is crucial that we also communicate and discuss our concerns with those people who are important to us. We need to give them an opportunity to express their worries and fears. Remember that your weight loss is not just happening to you. It is happening to your friends, your husband or wife, your children, and your family of origin. You may be tempted to think this is just your business. And it is primarily your business, but not completely so. Your weight loss is also impacting other people, and they will have feelings about it. It is not incumbent upon you to listen to or care about everyone's reaction to your change, but it is probably a good idea to care about the reactions of those closest to you. If your husband tells you that he is afraid you will leave him when you start getting attention from other men, it might be good for you to know that so you can allay his fears without necessarily succumbing to unreasonable demands on your freedom and autonomy. Having others validate your concerns while you validate theirs will go a long way toward smoothing over what can sometimes be a rocky relationship road back to a newly established stability.

Step 7. Brainstorming Alternate Ways of Coping with Emotions

Many of our interviewees realized only after the surgery that they tended to eat when they felt negative emotions. Some ate when they were sad; others ate when they were stressed out. These emotions did not simply disappear after the surgery. Some of them actually increased as the changes consequent to weight loss piled up. So now emotion was running high, and their habitual coping mechanism (eating) was no longer an option if they wanted to keep losing weight or maintain the loss. Becoming aware of these patterns prior to the surgery can be very helpful so that you don't get blindsided afterward.

- Identify the types of emotions that make you turn to food. You may be able to identify them immediately, or you may have to monitor yourself for a few weeks before surgery to figure out what characterizes those moments when you reach for food without even thinking about it. Having a diary in which you track these moments may be helpful. Clearly, you are going to have sad or frustrated or stressed-out moments after the surgery—for a little while, you might even have more of these as your life hangs in a state of flux.

- Compose a list of alternate ways in which you can self-soothe. This will come in very handy after the surgery. Eventually, you may learn to simply "surf" these emotions, which means that you let them come and go without feeling a need to react to them. Other folks need to replace eating with specific activities that serve a calming function. To one person that might be a bath, to another it might be lying down for a few minutes, and for yet another it may be playing with their dog. You will have to come up with your own customized list. It will also be helpful if that list is specific to different circumstances such as being home alone, at work, or at a party. Remember, though, that the types of coping activities you may conjure up in your presurgical brainstorming session may actually differ significantly from the ones you adopt after surgery. That is because prior to the surgery it probably will not occur to you to think of physical activity as a coping activity. Yet exercise will be a real possibility once the weight starts coming off. And exercise is a proven way to dissipate negative emotions and increase positive ones.

Step 8. Formalizing Current Self-Concept

How do you figure out what your current self-concept is? Very few of us ever engage in any exercise that tries to pinpoint what we actually think of ourselves: our strengths, our weaknesses, aspects of ourselves we think are situational versus those we think are essential and unchanging components of our nature. It can be very illuminating to do this in any situation because it makes us face the assumptions about ourselves under which we function.

⊙ Write down a description of who you think you are. List your good, bad, and neutral qualities. Some of the characteristics you will be able to trace to your past and messages you received from primary caregivers. "Johnny, you are not good at math!" "Mary, you are very disorganized!" Other qualities will feel so integral a part of you that you are convinced you would have exhibited them no matter who intervened. Other traits you will identify as ones that you worked very hard to develop and solidify. Make the list as long as you can. When you engage in this exercise you will find it hard to tease apart the way you view yourself from the way you think others see you. One of the reasons that it is useful to engage in this exercise is to realize that you really have a pretty formalized script for who you are and the role you play.

⊙ How do you feel about you? Much like a character in a screenplay, you have cast yourself in a role. The people in your life will also likely have cast you in a role. These roles may be very similar or quite different. The extent to which these roles feel congruent with the person you think you really are deep down or the extent to which those roles make you happy are up for assessment. And it is a very important assessment to conduct because the script can be rewritten to a surprising extent. Losing as much weight as you are likely to lose after obesity surgery will probably necessitate a script rewrite.

⊙ Who would you like to be? What aspects of who you are would you like to change? We go through much of our lives thinking that who we are is written in stone. But it isn't. We can make significant changes if we want to. A satisfying and functional rewrite of your script, however, requires that you know what the original version was. Knowing where you are is a prerequisite to charting a course to where you want to be.

Postsurgical Module

Step 9. Processing the Expectation-Reality Alignment

Six months to a year after surgery, you will find yourself having lost an enormous amount of weight. You will start to have an idea, though not yet complete, about which of your expectations seem to be in the process of being fulfilled, which ones do not even peek over the horizon, and which ones have already been fully met. This postsurgical assessment of the extent to which your expectations are aligning themselves with reality will be useful in a number of ways.

⊙ Is there anything you can do to bring reality more in alignment with your expectations? Maybe you need to work a little harder to make it happen. Maybe the weight loss is a facilitator, but you also need to pitch in with a different kind of elbow grease.

⊙ Which expectations are within your control and which aren't? Some things are very difficult to make happen. We all want to meet our perfect partner. We all want recognition for our achievements. Clearly, the attainment of these things is facilitated by our efforts, but sometimes our efforts are simply not sufficient. It is important to distinguish what is within your control and what isn't. It helps the emotional processing of the unfulfilled expectations outside of your control—some things you need to let go. It also helps you work harder on the ones you can influence. Maybe you are not everybody's dreamboat, even as a nonobese person. Or maybe you've come to realize that finding a good romantic relationship is hard, whether you're heavy or not.

⊚ Did your expectations aim high enough? Maybe your expectations were not ambitious enough. Maybe the weight loss has surpassed your most ambitious expectations and you need to calibrate those dreams to aim a little higher.

It is a good idea to monitor your level of satisfaction with the extent to which your expectations are coming true. You don't want disappointment or complacency sneaking in the back door and sabotaging your admirable efforts to change your life.

Step 10. Implementing Alternate Coping Strategies

Prior to the surgery, you brainstormed alternate ways to self-soothe when you started feeling bad about things. Now is the time to put these strategies to the test. You come home from a hard day at work, and your first impulse is to reach for the fridge door to munch on whatever is closest at hand. You are at home on a Saturday night wondering why the phone isn't ringing and why you still have no dates. Visions of Dairy Queen start dancing in your head. You are prepared for this. You knew it would happen, and you have a list of things to replace eating with, even if at this moment none of them sounds quite as alluring as these culinary temptations. You get up and you do them. No need to wonder what to do—you had planned for this ahead of time. It is also likely that you have now added to that alternate-coping-strategies list some exercise activities.

Revise your list of alternate coping strategies that replace emotional eating. Add activities to the list—ones you maybe didn't think of or couldn't do prior to the surgery. Early on in the process this may be a simple walk around the block, but as you get thinner, the exercise can be more entertaining, like tennis or aerobics or yoga. The bottom line is that these negative emotions can no longer surprise you with their call to eat; you have identified them, and you have a plan for dealing with them—a revised plan. That does not mean it will be effortless. Willpower will still have to rule, but it will have a much better chance of succeeding than if you had left the situation unexamined and ripe for the surprise attack of a bad day.

Step 11. Reconfiguring Self-concept

Once a month, you may want to revisit that self-concept script you wrote prior to the surgery. Does it still fit? Or does it need adjustments?

- Revise the list of characteristics that you think define who you are. You may find that you have to change some things about it every month. Write a revised copy and date it.

- Track which ones are changing and which ones are staying the same. It is a good idea to keep a copy of the original description, along with every monthly revision so that you can track your development.

The point here is that prior to the surgery, you started with the acknowledgment that your self-concept does not have to be rigid and set in stone. You bought into the idea that experiencing changes in self-concept does not have to be "crazy making," if you accept the idea that people change as a function of circumstance and will. Changes to that self-concept do not imply that you did not know who you were in the first place. It means that you understand that who you are is a work in progress. It means that you know you can change in response to changing feedback, without necessarily losing your center.

- Evaluate the extent to which you like or do not like the changes in who you are becoming. It is good to evaluate who you are becoming because you may need to redirect your development. Some of our interviewees expressed concern that the weight loss may have made them too self-focused at certain times. Charting that progress would make it easier to sit down and evaluate your feelings about the evolving you. This could lead to the enactments of adjustments in case you think the direction you are taking is not entirely desirable.

- Get feedback from significant others whom you trust and whom you judge not to be overly invested either way. You do run the risk of engendering conflict with this request if you do not have a high level of trust in the person you ask for feedback. It is always difficult to hear what others think of us, even when they are loved ones. If you do not feel up to it emotionally, don't ask. If you don't think there is someone in your life you trust this much, don't ask the wrong person. The point is you have to trust and respect the person you ask, and you have to be willing to truly hear the feedback in as nondefensive a fashion as possible.

Step 12. Practicing Social Skills and Appropriate Assertiveness

After the weight loss, you may find yourself engaged in social situations you are no longer accustomed to or never were. How should you act? What do you do when a waiter comes on to you? How do you respond to compliments? How does this dating thing work? When you have spent your life in a state of social avoidance, all of these new experiences may feel intimidating.

- Get information about what to do in certain situations. You can ask good friends, family members, members of a support group if you are attending one, or maybe a therapist or counselor if you have access to one.

- Practice these skills and role-play with trusted friends or with counselors and support-group members. You can also practice in front of a mirror and judge what feels right to you. It is unlikely that you are so off-base that you couldn't possibly get it right on your own.

- Develop your own style. You don't have to become someone you are not.

Ultimately, you will just have to go out there into the world and take your chances. Even without guidance, you will eventually figure out what works and what doesn't. The point is that you'll have to take some significant risks. The best attitude to adopt in these little risk sessions is "Okay, here I go! If it doesn't work, I may come across as awkward or unpolished or maybe even rude or aloof, but no one dies! I'll do it better next time." The alternative is to stay home and wither. That is, of course, no alternative at all.

The other aspect of social interaction that many of our interviewees struggled with was assertiveness. It is no doubt hard to go from self-effacement to appropriate requests. If you throw a little anger into the mix for all the years of having denied yourself or having been denied rightful consideration, aggressiveness can be the result. It isn't always easy to draw the line between being politely assertive and overbearingly pushy, even for folks who have not been obese. Again, this takes practice, and if you don't have people to practice with, trial and error should eventually work. It is important that you keep in mind that you are in a learning process and that you pay careful attention to feedback as a constructive force rather than as an insulting one.

Step 13. Communicating With Significant Others

As you go through all of this self-refection and skill building, it is important to keep significant people in your life apprised of your work and of some of the developments. This might be a confusing time for them also. The person they thought they knew so well starts to change before their very eyes, both physically and emotionally. It is not hard to understand why this might be disconcerting and fertile ground for misinterpretation. If you feel that your loved ones are essentially supportive of your attempts to improve your life, it is a good idea to keep them informed so that they know where you are coming from. It also sends the message that they are part of the journey.

- Communicate with your loved ones about the struggles you are confronting.

- Make gentle requests for readjustment in their behavior that would be helpful to your progress. These requests will be better met if the person knows the purpose of the adjustment and is not left to wonder if it is a threat to the relationship.

There will be times when conflict occurs regardless. This is to be expected when changes are taking place. Communicating openly, however, can only facilitate the resolution of the occasional disturbance. If all of this is taking place in the context of a support group or counseling, it may be very helpful to bring family members into the process from time to time. That way you can check in with their experience and perceptions of the ways in which the relationships are evolving throughout the weight loss process.

Step 14. Making Plans to Live Out Dreams

Once you have a more reality-tested idea of how your life is changing and of your potential without the shackles of obesity, it is time to make plans for those things you always wanted to do but believed were outside your reach.

- Make a list of your dreams—of the things you would like to accomplish. Some of these dreams may still be out of your reach, but a whole host of others will materialize on the horizon as real possibilities. They don't have to be huge plans, but they certainly can be. The dream can be about going to Disneyland with your kids, or it can be about going all out to try to make it as a recording artist. Whatever means something to you is good enough.

- Write a strategic plan of how you plan to work toward or accomplish these dreams. A number of our interviewees commented on how, long after the surgery and weight loss, they were still stuck in old patterns of thought. They often failed to realize what was now within the realm of the possible. They had become so accustomed to having no dreams that they had difficulty envisioning their desires, much less planning for ways of attaining them. Making a list can be very helpful—writing down systematic steps toward the fulfillment of these dreams can make them only more probable. Don't be afraid of jinxing anything by writing it down. You won't. The only jinx is not going for it.

Concluding Note

Neither Weight nor Weight Loss

Six years ago, thirty-three people sat down with us and graced us with their stories of how severe obesity and then weight loss had affected their lives. Their rich stories and impressions were about so much more than diets and pounds lost. They told a universal story of the complexity of human experience and how any attempt to reduce a life down to one component is no story at all. The real story of who they were was neither about weight nor weight loss. When these folks were severely obese, much of the world reduced them to their excess weight. They were the fat people. Their struggle to be heard and seen beyond the wall of their weight seemed mostly doomed to failure. Most were appalled at the world's inability to see them for anything other than their obesity. Upon meeting them, we too were appalled at what they had had to endure.

They were men and women who yearned to be loved and respected, who had children they worried about and careers they wanted to excel in. They then decided to do something about their weight and opted for obesity surgery. Although they had spent a lifetime either fighting or being disgusted by the idea that weight could determine who they were, they somewhat ironically invested weight loss with the power to change their lives. The discovery for most of them was that neither obesity nor weight loss defined them. Sure, most of their lives improved tremendously after the surgery, but they were still left with the existential struggle to define themselves, to take responsibility for their experiences, and to identify with both the freedom and the limitations of this life. In an essential way, isn't that everyone's story? It is, but they got to experience it with the heightened contrast of a very clear before-and-after experience. May we all learn from their tale, be we fat, thin, rich, poor, or simply trying to figure out who we are and who we want to be.

Selected Resources for Public and Health Professionals

Comprehensive Obesity Resources: Definitions, Causes, Prevalence, Advocacy, and Treatments of Obesity

American Obesity Association
1250 Twenty-fourth St. NW
Suite 300
Washington, DC 20037
Telephone: 202–776–7711
Fax: 202–776–7712
E-mail: executive@obesity.org
Web: http://www.obesity.org

SUMMARY: The American Obesity Association is devoted to advocacy and education on issues related to overweight and obesity. The comprehensive Web site promotes education, research, and community and government legislative action to improve the quality of life for people with obesity. Obesity fact sheets are available in Spanish.

Centers for Disease Control and Prevention
1600 Clifton Rd.
Atlanta, GA 30333
Public inquiries: 404–639–3534 or 800–311–3435
Web: http://www.cdc.gov/nccdphp/dnpa/obesity/

SUMMARY: The Department of Health and Human Services' Centers for Disease Control and Prevention offers a comprehensive collection of information and resources for individuals interested in learning more about overweight and obesity. The Web site contains the most recent statistics on the obesity epidemic, including a state-by-state graphical representation of obesity prevalence in the United States, definitions of overweight and obesity for adults and kids, economic consequences of obesity, information on improving nutrition and increasing physical activity, state-based programs, and frequently asked questions.

Obesity Action Coalition
4511 North Himes Ave.
Suite 250
Tampa, FL 33614
Telephone: 813–872–7835
Toll-free: 800–717–3117
Fax: 813–873–7838
E-mail: info@obesityaction.org
Web: http://www.obesityaction.org/

SUMMARY: The Obesity Action Coalition offers education, advocacy, and support to those affected by obesity and strives to eliminate the negative stigma associated with all types of obesity. Among numerous other features on their Web site are a body mass index calculator and a support-group locator by region.

ObesityHelp, Inc.
8001 Irvine Center Dr.
Suite 1270
Irvine, CA 92618
Telephone: 866–957–4636
Web: http://www.obesityhelp.com/home/

SUMMARY: ObesityHelp is dedicated to the education, empowerment, and support of all individuals affected by obesity, along with their families, friends, employers, surgeons, and physicians. It offers tools to locate professions by region and an opportunity to read reviews of their experiences, chat forums, and its own magazine. The Web site also features information on reconstructive surgery after weight loss surgery and a tool to help find a reconstructive surgeon by region.

Obesity Law and Advocacy Center
1392 East Palomar St.
Suite 403-233
Chula Vista, CA 91913
Telephone: 619-656-5251
Fax: 619-656-5254
Web: http://www.obesitylaw.com/

SUMMARY: The Obesity Law and Advocacy Center provides advocacy for morbidly obese persons who have been denied health insurance coverage for medically necessary procedures or who have been wrongfully terminated or discriminated against in the workplace because of their weight.

Weight-Control Information Network
1 WIN Way
Bethesda, MD 20892-3665
Phone: 202-828-1025
Toll-free: 877-946-4627
Fax: 202-828-1028
E-mail: WIN@info.niddk.nih.gov
Web: http://www.win.niddk.nih.gov

SUMMARY: The Weight-Control Information Network (WIN) is a service of the National Institute of Diabetes and Digestive and Kidney Diseases of the National Institutes of Health, which is the U.S. government's lead agency responsible for biomedical research on nutrition and obesity. Authorized by Congress (Public Law 103-43), WIN provides the general public, health professionals, the media, and Congress with up-to-date, science-based information on weight control, obesity, physical activity, and related nutritional issues.

Weight Loss–Surgery Books

Apple, R. F., J. Locke, and R. Peeples. *Preparing for Weight Loss Surgery Workbook.* New York: Oxford University Press, 2006.
Goldberg, M. C., G. Cowan, and W. Y. Marcus. *Weight Loss Surgery: Is It Right for You?* New York: Square One Publishers, 2005.
Janeway, J. M., K. J. Sparks, and R. S. Baker. *The Real Skinny on Weight Loss Surgery:*

An Indispensable Guide to What You Can Really Expect! Onondaga, Mich.: Little Victories Press, 2005.

Kurian, M. S., B. Thompson, and B. K. Davidson. *Weight Loss Surgery for Dummies.* New York: Wiley, 2005.

Woodward, B. G. *A Complete Guide to Obesity Surgery: Everything You Need to Know About Weight Loss Surgery and How to Succeed.* Victoria, B.C.: Trafford, 2001.

Nutrition and Physical Fitness Resources

For information about the new food pyramid, visit the U.S. Department of Agriculture's Web site at http://www.mypyramid.gov. For information about understanding and using the "Nutrition Facts" label on food products, visit the U.S. Food and Drug Administration's Web site at http://www.cfsan.fda .gov/~dms/foodlab.html. For an overview of bariatric dietary guidelines, go to http://www.obesityaction.org/resources/oacnews/oacnews2/nutrition.php.

For postoperative weight loss–surgery recipes, see the following sources:

Furtado, M., and L. Schultz. *Recipes for Life After Weight-Loss Surgery: Delicious Dishes for Nourishing the New You.* Beverly, Mass.: Fair Winds Press, 2007.

Levine, P., M. Bontmpo-Saray, W. B. Inabnet, and M. Urban-Skuros. *Eating Well After Weight Loss Surgery: Over 140 Delicious Low-Fat, High-Protein Recipes to Enjoy in the Weeks, Months and Years After Surgery.* New York: Marlowe, 2004.

Information and Clinical Guidelines for Bariatric Professionals

American Society of Bariatric Physicians
2821 S. Parker Rd.
Suite 625
Aurora, CO 80014
Automated Referral Line: 303–779–4833
Fax: 303–779–4834
E-mail: bariatric@asbp.org
Web: http://www.asbp.org

SUMMARY: The American Society of Bariatric Physicians (ASBP) is a professional medical society of licensed physicians who specialize in the medical treatment of obesity (bariatrics) and its associated conditions. The society offers practical information for medical doctors and the general public and supports public policies to prevent overweight and obesity. The ASBP also provides tips on weight loss and a referral program to reach member physicians for professional consultation.

American Society for Metabolic and Bariatric Surgery
100 SW Seventy-fifth Street
Suite 201
Gainesville, FL 32607
Telephone: 352–331–4900
Fax: 352–331–4975
E-mail: info@asmbs.org
Web: http://www.asmbs.org

SUMMARY: The American Society for Metabolic and Bariatric Surgery is dedicated to the advancement of bariatric surgery. The society provides information on obesity, bariatric surgery, and related topics to professionals and the public. The Web site contains the 1994 consensus statement of the ASMBS, names and contact information of doctors who specialize in bariatric surgery, and suggestions for the presurgical psychological assessment of bariatric-surgery candidates.

North American Association for the Study of Obesity
8630 Fenton St.
Suite 918
Silver Spring, MD 20910
Telephone: 301–563–6526
Fax: 301–563–6595
Web: http://www.naaso.org

SUMMARY: NAASO, the Obesity Society, is the leading scientific society dedicated to the study of obesity. The Obesity Society promotes research, education, and advocacy to better understand, prevent, and treat obesity and improve the lives of those affected. The Obesity Society is committed to encouraging research on the causes and treatment of obesity and to keeping the medical community and public informed of new advances. The Obesity Society's official journal, *Obesity,* publishes original scientific articles, as well as relevant review articles, commentaries, and public health and medical news.

For clinicians treating clinically severely obese individuals, see the following helpful books and resources.

Apple, R. F., J. Locke, and R. Peeples. *Preparing for Weight Loss Surgery: Therapists Guide.* New York: Oxford University Press, 2006.

Fairburn, C. G. *Overcoming Binge Eating.* New York: Guilford Press, 1995.

Fairburn, C. G., and K. D. Brownell, eds. *Eating Disorder and Obesity: A Comprehensive Handbook.* 2d ed. New York: Guilford Press, 2002.

Mitchell, J. E., and M. de Zwaan, eds. *Bariatric Surgery: Psychosocial Assessment and Treatment.* New York: Brunner/Mazel, 2005.

Practical Guide to the Identification, Evaluation and Treatment of Overweight and Obesity in Adults: Clinical Guidelines on the Identification, Evaluation, and Treatment of Overweight and Obesity in Adults. 1998. Retrieved from the National Institutes of Health, National Heart, Lung, and Blood Institute's Web site at http://www.nhlbi.nih.gov/guidelines/obesity/.

Notes

Introduction

1. Data from the Healthcare Cost and Utilization Project Nationwide Inpatient Sample indicate that the death rate among weight loss–surgery patients as a whole fell by 64 percent, from 0.89 percent to 0.32 percent between 1998 and 2002. This represents a decrease from nine to three deaths per every one thousand surgeries. See W. Encinosa et al., "Use and Costs of Bariatric Surgery and Prescription Weight-Loss Medications."

2. According to the Centers for Disease Control and Prevention's Web site, 65 percent of adults (twenty years or older) were classified as overweight (body mass index [BMI] of 25 or greater) between the years 1999 and 2002. Additionally, 31 percent were classified as obese (BMI equal to or greater than 30), and 4.7 percent were considered clinically severely obese (BMI greater than or equal to 40). Data are based on the 2002 National Health and Nutrition Examination Survey. These and more data are available in C. L. Ogden et al., "Mean Body Weight, Height, and Body Mass Index, United States, 1960–2002."

3. The American Society for Metabolic and Bariatric Surgery estimates that 170,000 surgeries were performed in the 2005. This figure was obtained from Julie Nichols, continuing medical education coordinator, American Society for Metabolic and Bariatric Surgery, October 31, 2006, via a personal e-mail. According to a 2005 article published in the *Archives of Surgery,* the number of weight loss surgeries performed in the United States between 1998 and 2002 increased 450 percent (from 12,775 to 70,256 cases). For more data and information, see N. T. Nguyen et al., "Accelerated Growth of Bariatric Surgery With the Introduction of Minimally Invasive Surgery"; and W. J. Pories and G. M. Pratt, "Commentary: Quality Control of Bariatric Surgery."

4. There was a 144 percent increase in the number of American Society for Metabolic and Bariatric Surgery (ASMBS) bariatric surgeons, and a 146 percent increase in the number of bariatric centers. According to the ASMBS, there were more than 140,000 bariatric procedures performed in 2004, nearly double the

number during the year 2002. See Nguyen et al., "Accelerated Growth"; and Pories and Pratt, "Commentary."

5. Nearly all disciplines within the field of surgery are being revolutionized by minimally invasive surgery techniques. Laparoscopic procedures are now widely used to perform all types of weight loss surgeries. The University of Chicago Center for Surgical Treatment of Obesity maintains an informative Web site describing laparoscopy (http://www.uchospitals.edu/specialties/minisurgery/mis .html).

6. For a more detailed discussion regarding the various types of weight loss surgeries that are currently being performed, visit the ASMBS Web site (http://www .asmbs.org.) or that of ObesityHelp (http://www.obesityhelp.com). Additionally, *Weight Loss Surgery for Dummies* by M. S. Kurian, B. Thompson, and B. K. Davidson provides a general overview of the various bariatric surgery options.

7. Dietary guidelines after surgery typically vary somewhat depending on the specific bariatric program and the type of surgery. The fundamental principles of these postoperative bariatric diets, however, are essentially the same. For example, most programs encourage patients (regardless of surgery type) to consume their protein first, to avoid drinking liquids during meals, and to eat very slowly. An excellent overview of bariatric dietary guidelines can be found on the Obesity Action Coalition's Web site (http://www.obesityaction.org/resources/oacnews/ oacnews2/nutrition.php).

8. Hospital discharge data extracted from the Nationwide Inpatient Sample between the years 1996 and 2002 revealed that although the rates of bariatric surgery in the overall sample increased more than sevenfold during the study period, the proportion of bariatric surgery patients who were female remained constant, between 81.5 percent and 85.3 percent. See M. M. Davis et al., "National Trends in Bariatric Surgery, 1996–2002."

9. There is a substantial body of literature consistently showing that women utilize health care services more frequently than men. A fairly recent study by K. D. Bertakis and colleagues, "Gender Differences in the Utilization of Health Care Services" (2000), found that utilization of medical services and associated health care costs remained significantly higher for women even when controlling for health status and other demographic variables, such as socioeconomic status. At present, it appears that the explanation for these gender discrepancies is somewhat complex and multifaceted. For example, some theorists attribute the differences to women seeking services for female-specific conditions, such as issues related to reproductive biology, whereas others point to gender differences in willingness to report symptoms and illnesses.

10. There is no question that there is tremendous prejudice toward obese in-

dividuals. It is now becoming increasingly apparent that the stigma facing obese persons is generally greater for women than for men. Greater bias and stigmatization among obese women compared to obese men have been demonstrated in the selection of desired sexual partners, hiring practices of potential employers, workplace compensation, and college admittance. Additionally, more women than men have reported experiencing perceived weight-related discrimination. For a comprehensive overview of weight-related discrimination, see E. Y. Chen and M. Brown, "Obesity Stigma in Sexual Relationships"; N. H. Falkner et al., "Mistreatment Due to Weight: Prevalence and Sources of Perceived Mistreatment in Women and Men"; and R. Puhl and K. D. Brownell, "Bias, Discrimination, and Obesity."

11. For those interested in more detail on grounded-theory methodology in qualitative research, see K. Chamberlain, "Using Grounded Theory in Health Psychology: Practices, Premises, and Potential."

12. See L. E. Bocchieri, M. Meana, and B. L. Fisher, "Perceived Psychosocial Outcomes of Gastric Bypass Surgery: A Qualitative Study."

13. See L. Bocchieri-Ricciardi et al., "Investigation of Weight-Related Relationship Adjustment in Female Obesity Surgery Patients"; L. Bocchieri, M. Meana, and B. L. Fisher, "Perceived Psychosocial Outcomes of Gastric Bypass Surgery: A Qualitative Investigation," "The Question of Outcomes in Gastric Bypass Surgery," and "Sexual Functioning Following Gastric Bypass Surgery: A Qualitative Investigation."

Chapter 1. Taking the Leap: Deciding on Surgery

1. The data summarizing the five out of ten leading causes of death that are directly linked to obesity can be found in F. Berg, *Health Risks of Obesity*. In addition, the American Obesity Association's Web site maintains a comprehensive fact sheet outlining all of the medical conditions associated with obesity (http://www .obesity.org/subs/fastfacts/Health_Effects.shtml).

2. For a comprehensive review of the numerous character flaws ascribed to obese persons, see Puhl and Brownell, "Bias, Discrimination, and Obesity."

3. A. J. Stunkard and T. I. Sorensen refer to the discrimination against obese individuals as a prejudice that many in the general public don't even feel compelled to hide. They refer to it as "one of the last acceptable forms of prejudice." For an illuminating article on the topic, see Stunkard and Sorenson, "Obesity and Socioeconomic Status: A Complex Relation."

4. Numerous studies have documented the early development in children of negative attitudes toward the obese. One study by P. Cramer and T. Steinwert (1998)

suggests that negative attitudes toward obese persons are evident in children as young as three years old ("Thin Is Good, Fat Is Bad: How Early Does It Begin?"). Other studies include C. R. Counts et al., "The Perception of Obesity by Normal-Weight Versus Obese School-Age Children"; S. A. Richardson et al., "Cultural Uniformity in Reaction to Physical Disabilities"; and J. R. Staffieri, "A Study of Social Stereotype of Body Image in Children."

5. Some evolutionary theorists have proposed that human beings may be biologically predisposed to make distinctions between groups. It has been hypothesized that harboring feelings of attachment to one group and animosity for another group might have been a strategy that facilitated survival. It would mean that one group would hoard resources for their genetic kin and thus promote their survival. For a discussion of evolutionary theory and discrimination, see H. D. Fishbein, *Peer Prejudice and Discrimination: Evolutionary, Cultural, and Developmental Dynamics.*

6. An investigation of college applications during the 1960s by H. Canning and J. Mayer found that regardless of equivalent application rates and academic performance, obese applicants were significantly less likely to be accepted to college compared to their nonobese peers ("Obesity: Its Possible Effect on College Acceptance"). M. V. Roehling published a comprehensive review of discrimination toward obese individuals in the workplace ("Weight-Based Discrimination in Employment: Psychological and Legal Aspects"). And negative attitudes and beliefs of health care workers toward obese patients have been documented across numerous studies and found to exist among physicians, nurses, dieticians, and medical students. Biased attitudes and beliefs toward the obese impact the delivery of medical and psychological services and affect the extent to which obese persons seek medical treatment when needed. See R. Hoppe and J. Ogden, "Practice Nurses' Beliefs About Obesity and Weight-Related Interventions in Primary Care"; M. Keane, "Contemporary Beliefs About Mental Illness Among Medical Students: Implications for Education and Practice"; D. Klein et al., "Patient Characteristics That Elicit Negative Responses From Family Physicians"; and L. McArthur and J. Ross, "Attitudes of Registered Dietitians Toward Personal Overweight and Overweight Clients."

7. Based on the available evidence examining the effectiveness of behavior modification and drug therapy for obesity, the National Institute Consensus Conference on the Surgery of Obesity in 1991 concluded that weight loss surgery is the only effective therapy for clinically severe obesity. These recommendations still stand today. For more information, visit http://www.nih.gov. Additionally, for a review of the nonsurgical approaches to obesity treatment, see A. J. Stunkard, "Current Views of Obesity."

8. A couple of references that detail the difficulty in weight loss and weight

loss maintenance are M. K. Serdula et al., "Prevalence of Attempting Weight Loss and Strategies for Controlling Weight"; and Technology Assessment Conference Statement, "Methods for Voluntary Weight Loss and Control."

9. Surveys of patients attending surgery clinics suggest that most patients are relatively well informed, although there are a minority who are not. In any case, there seems to be a professional near consensus that being well informed about the surgery is important to outcomes. In one survey of obesity surgery clinics nationwide, it was found that 70 percent of clinics considered lack of information about obesity surgery to be a contraindication for surgery. See A. U. Bauchowitz et al., "Psychosocial Evaluation of Bariatric Surgery Candidates: A Survey of Current Practices"; and T. A. Wadden and D. B. Sarwer, "Behavioral Assessment of Candidates for Bariatric Surgery: A Patient-Oriented Approach."

10. Health research into effective interventions to stop injurious behavior has repeatedly shown that scaring people with the health consequences of a behavior is not always effective. Smoking cessation is a specific example of how merely presenting the consequences of smoking has little to no impact on said behavior, largely because most people already know the risks associated with the behavior. In the case of cigarettes, the health risks are even printed on every pack. See J. W. McKenna and K. N. Williams, "Crafting Effective Tobacco Counter-Advertisements: Lessons From a Failed Campaign Directed at Teenagers."

11. Doctors advising patients to take action in regard to certain health behaviors has shown to facilitate health behavior change. Two areas in which doctor recommendations have been shown to have an impact are mammography use and smoking cessation. See B. K. Rimer, "Understanding the Acceptance of Mammography by Women"; and T. E. Kottke et al., "Attributes of Successful Smoking Cessation Interventions in Medical Practice: A Meta-analysis of 39 Controlled Trials."

12. See J. O. Prochaska and W. F. Velicer, "The Transtheoretical Model of Health Behavior Change."

13. In 1967, J. B. Overmeier and M. E. P. Seligman coined the term *learned helplessness* to describe the state in which people (and animals) learn to be helpless when they experience a lack of control over negative circumstances. In Overmeier and Seligman's seminal study, dogs who had been repeatedly conditioned to expect an inescapable shock after a bell tone eventually stopped trying to escape after the bell was rung—even when given the opportunity to do so easily. The dogs had learned previously that nothing they did mattered. They had learned that they could not escape the inevitable shock—and so they sat passively and helplessly. Later studies revealed that learned helplessness was associated with depressive symptoms, and thus the concept became a model for explaining depression. The learned-helplessness model of depression remains an important piece of the depression puzzle today; however, it has been reformulated

to include aspects of attribution theory (how one explains certain events). See Overmeier and Seligman, "Effects of Inescapable Shock Upon Subsequent Escape and Avoidance Responding"; and C. Petersen, S. F. Maier, and M. E. P. Seligman, *Learned Helplessness: A Theory for the Age of Personal Control.*

14. A. Keys et al., *The Biology of Human Starvation.*

15. For a sense of the caloric intake in popular diets, see H. M. Wim. Saris, "Very Low-Calorie Diets and Sustained Weight Loss."

16. There are differences of opinion about what constitutes an addiction. Some purists argue that addictions need to involve the ingestion of a substance that alters the individual's experience of themselves or of their environment. Lately, however, arguments are being made that behaviors such as eating or sex can rise to the level of addictions. For a discussion of this controversy, see P. R. Martin and N. Petry, "Are Non-Substance-Related Addictions Really Addictions?"

17. The National Institute of Mental Health offers a downloadable (PDF) booklet describing the symptoms, causes, and treatments for depression with information on getting help and coping (http://www.nimh.nih.gov/publicat/depression.cfm).

18. Many individuals suffering from depression have improved their symptoms via the self-help approach. There are numerous self-help depression books on the market today. Two that we commonly recommend to our clients are D. Burns, *The Feeling Good Handbook;* and D. Greenberger and C. A. Padesky, *Mind Over Mood: Change How You Feel by Changing the Way You Think.* The self-help approach is particularly useful when limited mobility or inability to pay for therapy interfere with engaging in outpatient psychotherapy. Additionally, these books are often used in conjunction with face-to-face psychotherapy.

Chapter 2. Responding to the Kindness of Strangers: Now You Don't See Me, Now You Do

1. For more information regarding the common behaviors (warning signs) of those with eating disorders, visit the National Eating Disorders Association's Web site (http://www.nationaleatingdisorders.org).

2. Studies have routinely demonstrated that body dissatisfaction tends to be significantly higher in women than it is in men, particularly in relation to body weight. Body-image dissatisfaction has also been linked to decreased self-esteem. Studies that have investigated gender differences and the relationship between body dissatisfaction and self-esteem include S. C. Abell and M. H. Richards, "The Relationship Between Body Shape Satisfaction and Self-esteem: An Investigation of Gender and Class Differences"; and M. Tiggeman, "Body-Size Dissatisfaction: Individual Differences in Age and Gender and Relationship With Self-esteem."

3. For a review of perceptions of obese individuals, see R. Puhl and K. D. Brownell, "Bias, Discrimination, and Obesity.

4. *Resiliency* is a term used in psychology to describe the capacity of people to deal with stress in adaptive ways. There appear to be individual differences in resiliency, with some folks able to cope with significant hardship, whereas others become significantly more incapacitated. In recent years, a great deal of research has been devoted to the concept of resiliency. For an interesting scientific review on the topic of resiliency, see M. D. Resnick, "Protective Factors, Resiliency, and Healthy Youth Development."

5. Some people object to the use of the term *opposite sex* because (1) they believe it sets up an adversarial relationship between men and women, (2) it fails to include individuals who do not identify exclusively as males or females, such as some transsexual and intersex individuals, and (3) it lends support to a restrictive view of the world as consisting of only two sexes or genders despite the existence of individuals who do not fit neatly into this system. Although the authors are sympathetic to all efforts that make language as inclusive and nonadversarial as possible, there is no clearer term when speaking of heterosexual men and women. Thus, we have maintained the use of "opposite sex," while here acknowledging that it is a compromise in the service of clarity and not meant to exclude any individuals or support any system of thought that does so.

6. Some theorists believe that being an object of desire is part of the female gender role for biological and evolutionary reasons, whereas others think that our society consistently objectifies women and traps them in this "object of desire" role. There is probably a combination of both forces at play. For arguments on both sides of the debate, see B. Ellis and D. Symons, "Sex Differences in Sexual Fantasy: An Evolutionary Psychological Approach"; and B. Fredrickson and T. Roberts, "Objectification Theory."

7. In 1994, using state-of-the-art sampling procedures, the National Opinion Research Center at the University of Chicago conducted a large-scale procedures survey investigating the sexual practices of Americans. The survey found that 12 percent of women and 23 percent of men had engaged in extramarital sex. See M. W. Weiderman, "Extramarital Sex: Prevalence and Correlates in a National Survey."

Chapter 3. Changing the Dynamics in Your Inner Circle: Your Change Becomes Everybody Else's

1. The formal theory that best accounts for the interconnectedness of relationships is family systems theory. It is a theory of human behavior based on the

ecological principle that human beings do not live in isolation and can be better understood when viewed within the context of dynamic, interconnected human interactions and relationships. For a brief overview of family systems theory on the Internet, see "Overview of Biopsychosocial Theories; Socially Oriented Theories: Family Systems," chap. 3 of *Psychological Self-Tools: Online Self-Help Book,* http://mentalhelp.net/poc/view_doc.php?type=doc&id=9717&cn=353. For a more comprehensive overview of systems therapy and applications in clinical practice, see M. Bowen, *Family Therapy in Clinical Practice.*

2. Health psychologists have long observed that being ill or engaging in illness behavior (and we don't mean faking illness) often brings secondary gains (a term coined by Freud). Secondary gains are defined as the rewards or benefits of the sick role. These gains can include attention, sympathy, or relief from responsibilities. Most people don't even realize that there are "benefits" to being sick, and many would be offended by the suggestion. But the concept of secondary gain does not imply that people enjoy being sick—it simply raises the issue that some bad situations have hidden rewards. Needless to say, the gains from being ill are nowhere near as significant as the losses. For an excellent review of the scientific evidence supporting the concept of secondary gain, see D. A. Fishbain et al., "Secondary Gain Concept: A Review of the Scientific Evidence."

3. There is a significant body of literature suggesting that the symptom of obesity can be conceptualized to exist as part of the larger system of the family. This family systems perspective suggests that relationship patterns contribute to the etiology and maintenance of obesity, and, in turn, the symptom of obesity maintains the system of the relationship. See L. Fishmann-Havstad and A. R. Marston, "Weight Loss as an Aspect of Family Emotion and Process"; R. M. Ganley, "Epistemology, Family Patterns, and Psychosomatics: The Case of Obesity"; J. E. Harkaway, "Obesity: Reducing the Larger System"; and R. B. Stuart and B. Jacobson, *Weight, Sex, and Marriage: A Delicate Balance.*

4. There have been few studies investigating marital quality and satisfaction before and after surgery. Of these studies, the results have been mixed. In one particular study by C. S. W. Rand, K. Kowalske, and J. M. Kuldau, "Characteristics of Marital Improvement Following Obesity Surgery," obesity surgery resulted in an overall decrease in marital conflict at one year. Interestingly, though, the rate of divorce was higher for the surgery patients than for comparison adults, particularly in marriages that were rated as conflicted prior to surgery. Thus, it seems that marital improvements were in no way universal. The following studies have also reported general improvements in marital quality after surgery: C. S. W. Rand, J. M. Kuldau, and L. Robbins, "Surgery for Obesity and Marriage Quality"; and S. L. Dubovsky et al., "A Preliminary Study of the Relationship

Between Preoperative Depression and Weight Loss Following Surgery for Morbid Obesity."

5. Using various methodologies, several studies have reported an increase in marital conflict or an overall deterioration in marriages after surgical weight loss. For more detailed information about some of these studies, see R. J. Hafner, "Morbid Obesity: Effects on the Marital System of Weight Loss After Gastric Restriction"; J. R. Marshall and J. Neill, "The Removal of a Psychosomatic Symptom: Effects on the Marriage"; and J. R. Neill, J. R. Marshall, and C. E. Yale, "Marital Changes After Intestinal Bypass Surgery."

6. L. C. Porter and R. S. Wampler conducted the most recent prospective study directly investigating postsurgical marital change ("Adjustment to Rapid Weight Loss"). Using standardized measures of depression, marital adjustment, and self-esteem, the authors assessed vertical-banded gastroplasty patients preoperatively and at six and twelve months. The results of this study are interesting in that there was an overall decrease in depression and an increase in self-esteem. However, overall results of the Locke-Wallace Marital Adjustment Test (MAT) yielded no significant change in marital satisfaction. On closer examination, it appears that the range of change in MAT scores was actually quite large and that the distribution tended toward bimodality, with some patients reporting an increase in marital adjustment and others reporting a significant decrease. These results support the contention that surgical weight loss has variable effects on marriage.

7. Data from the University of Chicago suggest that clinically and statistically significant improvements in quality of life, self-esteem, and depression can be detected as early as two to four weeks after surgery. See M. P. Dymek et al., "Quality of Life After Gastric Bypass Surgery: A Cross-sectional Study."

8. The term *self-efficacy* refers to people's beliefs about their ability to exercise control in order to affect their lives. However, self-efficacy is a specific rather than a global concept, which means that you can have high self-efficacy in one area and low self-efficacy in another. This concept was introduced to the field of psychology by Albert Bandura, and it has been an important one, especially in regards to health behavior. If people do not have high self-efficacy for a certain health behavior, such as breast self-examination, then they are unlikely to engage in this behavior. The same goes for smoking cessation or weight loss. If self-efficacy for accomplishing any of these is low, then health professionals need to invest in raising the public's self-efficacy with instructional materials and other resources. One of Bandura's articles in which he elaborated on the concept of self-efficacy is "Human Agency in Social Cognitive Theory."

9. Research with both children and adults confirms a consistent gender difference in temperament and in the prevalence of specific categories of emotional

problems. In childhood, girls are more prone to display inhibitory control than boys, and, in adulthood, women are more prone to internalizing disorders, such as depression and anxiety. Men are more prone to externalizing disorders such as those involving antisocial behavior and substance abuse. It has been suggested that maybe this gender difference lies in the different emphasis placed by men and women on the self versus the collective or group. Two references relating to this intriguing gender difference and N. M. Else-Quest et al., "Gender Differences in Temperament: A Meta-analysis"; and S. Rosenfield, M. C. Lennon, and H. R. White, "The Self and Mental Health: Self-salience and the Emergence of Internalizing and Externalizing Problems."

10. Studies that have investigated changes in sexuality after weight loss generally suggest positive results. Although there are reports of decreased sexual functioning following surgery, most studies have found the physical aspects of sex to be more enjoyable. On improvements in sexual relations after weight loss surgery, see E. E. Abramson and S. Catalano, "Weight Loss and Sexual Behavior"; M. A. Camps et al., "Impact of Bariatric Surgery on Body Image Perception and Sexuality in Morbidly Obese Patients and Their Partners"; P. Castelnuovo-Tedesco et al., "Long-term Outcome of Jejuno-ileal Bypass Surgery for Superobesity: A Psychiatric Assessment"; P. Chandarana et al., "Psychosocial Considerations in Gastric Stapling Surgery"; and L. K. Goble, C. S. W. Rand, and J. M. Kuldau, "Understanding Marital Relationships Following Obesity Surgery."

11. After surgery, the majority of patients report that the physical aspects of sex become easier and more pleasurable. A few studies have reported an emergence of sexual problems that did not exist prior to surgery with some patients experiencing decreased functioning or desire after surgery. Some reasons cited for worsened sexual functioning in these studies include decreased body image as a result of excess skin, reevaluation of sexual partners (they no longer seemed as attractive) after surgery, and spousal conflict. See L. E. Bocchieri, M. Meana, and B. L. Fisher, "Sexual Functioning Following Gastric Bypass Surgery: A Qualitative Investigation"; H. Hey and U. Niebuhr-Jorgensen, "Jejuno-ileal Bypass Surgery in Obesity: Gynecological and Obstetrical Aspects"; and J. F. Kinzl et al., "Partnership, Sexuality, and Sexual Disorders in Morbidly Obese Women: Consequence of Weight Loss After Gastric Banding."

12. The largest epidemiological study of sexual behavior in North America revealed that women rate their sexual satisfaction as high even when they are having problems with desire, arousal, and orgasm. This confusing finding seems to indicate that women claim they are relatively satisfied with their sexual relationship as long as they are satisfied with other aspects of their relationship with their partner. It may be an indication of the greater importance that women tend to

place on general relationship quality than on the actual quality of sexual inter-actions. It may also mean that they do not perceive their sexual problems as a function of anything that their partner is doing wrong, but rather as some aspect of themselves. It is a consistent and intriguing finding. To review the findings of this large study of sexual behavior in men and women in the United States, see E. O. Laumann et al., *The Social Organization of Sexuality: Sexual Practices in the United States.*

13. ObesityHelp provides a brief overview of reconstructive surgery for bar-iatric patients who are bothered by excess skin. See their Website (http://www .obesityhelp.com/content/lifeafter.html). This site also offers patients reviews of plastic surgeons who perform postbariatric reconstructive surgery and tools to locate a plastic surgeon by region.

14. Levels of estrogen and testosterone have been positively linked to body mass index in women, which may in part explain the positive associations be-tween obesity and breast cancer risk. When women lose massive amounts of weight, their estrogen and testosterone levels are likely to drop. For a recent sci-entific study linking estrogen to weight, see A. McTiernan et al., "Relation of BMI and Physical Activity to Sex Hormones in Post-menopausal Women."

15. The link between testosterone and sexual desire is stronger than that of es-trogen and sexual desire. There is also accumulating evidence that testosterone impacts sexual desire in surgically menopausal women. It remains important, however, to note that no single estrogen or testosterone level has been found predictive of low desire in either sex. The following studies provide data to sup-port this statement: G. Bachman et al., "Female Androgen Insufficiency: The Princeton Consensus Statement on Definition, Classification, and Assessment"; S. R. Davis et al., "Circulating Androgen Levels and Self-reported Sexual Function in Women"; R. C. Schiavi et al., "Effect of Testosterone Administration on Sexual Behavior and Mood in Men With Erectile Dysfunction"; and J. L. Shifren et al., "Transdermal Testosterone Treatment in Women With Impaired Sexual Function After Oopherectomy."

Chapter 4. Deconstructing the Self: Who Was I and Who Am I Becoming?

1. Although most people walk around thinking that their personalities have essentially developed as a product of their experiences in life, there are very convincing data indicating that certain broadly drawn personality traits may be mostly inherited. That is not to say that the environment has no impact on our personalities, but we seem to be relatively predisposed toward certain broad patterns of emotional processing and behaving. See R. Plomin et al., *Behavioral*

Genetics; and B. W. Roberts and W. F. DelVecchio, "The Rank-Order Consistency of Personality Traits From Childhood to Old-Age: A Quantitative Review of Longitudinal Studies."

2. The influence of genetics on obesity is well established. Many of the sources in "Selected Resources for the Public and Health Professionals" have information about the genetic component of obesity. The following article provides an interesting way to calculate an individual patient's genetic obesity risk: R. C. Thirlby and J. Randall, "A Genetic 'Obesity Risk Index' for Patients With Morbid Obesity."

3. Researchers at the Yale Eating and Weight Disorders Clinic have compiled a compelling argument that rapid acceleration of obesity in recent years can be attributed to the food industry and our increasingly sedentary behavior. See K. D. Brownell and K. B. Horgen, *Food Fight.*

4. Superobese individuals (BMI>60) may experience a higher rate of complications and mortality when compared to less obese patients, following bariatric surgery. This seems to be particularly true when the surgical approach is laparoscopic. For this reason, some surgeons will insist on weight loss prior to surgery, whereas others will even consider patients who are superobese as inoperable due to the unacceptably high risks involved. Weight loss failures (lowest postsurgical BMI>35) are also more common in this group of patients. Several studies that have investigated this issue include J. C. Gould et al., "Laparoscopic Gastric Bypass: Risk vs. Benefits up to Two Years Following Surgery in Super-Super Obese Patients"; L. D. MacLean, B. M. Rhode, and C. W. Nohr, "Late Outcomes of Isolated Gastric Bypass"; D. Oliak et al., "Short-term Results of Laparoscopic Gastric Bypass in Patients With BMI >60"; and H. J. Sugerman et al., "Weight Loss With Vertical Banded Gastroplasty and Roux-Y Gastric Bypass for Morbid Obesity With Selective Versus Random Assignment."

5. There are scientists who study the way people structure and process information. One of the ideas that has developed out of these efforts is the concept of a schema. A schema refers to an organized set of beliefs each individual has about a number of areas. We have schemas about relationships, about age, and about who we are, just to name a few. We may even have a schema about weight. One of the pioneers in schema theory actually studied weight schemas. A couple of references relating to self schemas and to weight include H. Markus, "Self-Schemata and Processing Information About the Self"; and H. Markus, R. Hamill, and K. P. Sentis, "Thinking Fat: Self Schemas for Body Weight and the Processing of Weight-Relevant Information."

6. The following are two reviews on body-image distortions in eating disorders: T. Cash and E. A. Deagle, "The Nature and Extent of Body-Image Disturbances in Anorexia Nervosa and Bulimia Nervosa: A Meta-analysis"; and S. Skrzypek,

P. M. Wehmeier, and H. Remschmidt, "Body Image Assessment Using Body Size Estimation in Recent Studies on Anorexia Nervosa: A Brief Review."

7. Whenever a group is stigmatized and discriminated against, the members of that stigmatized group can end up believing the negative things that are communicated about them. These stigmatized groups, be they women, ethnic minority groups, sexual minority groups, or severely obese individuals, will internalize the prejudice and the discrimination. Often, folks are not aware that they have done it or that they are in the process of doing it. It is a very common and injurious consequence of prejudice and discrimination.

Chapter 5. Facing the Music of Self:
When Weight Is No Longer the Reason

1. For a good review of the most common obesity surgeries performed today as well as their potential complications, see M. L. Kendrick and G. F. Dakin, "Surgical Approaches to Obesity."

2. Binge eating is commonly considered to be an uncontrolled reaction to negative emotions. Emotional eating is then assumed to make individuals feel better and to serve as a distraction from these negative affective states. It is generally considered a form of avoidance coping wherein the individual eats to avoid feeling or expressing emotions that are disturbing. Much has been written on the link between eating and emotion. For an excellent review on the risk factors for eating pathology, see E. Stice, "Risk and Maintenance Factors for Eating Pathology: A Meta-analytic Review."

3. See American Psychiatric Association Work Group on Eating Disorders, "Practice Guidelines for the Treatment of Patients With Eating Disorders (Revision)"; and R. L. Spitzer et al., "Binge-Eating Disorder: Its Further Validation in a Multisite Study."

4. Many clinicians and researchers have noted that individuals with a history of child and adult sexual abuse blame themselves for the sexual encounters. They commonly attribute the abuse to some deficiency in themselves rather than in the perpetrator. This makes for feelings of shame and guilt and adds to the emotional distress around the trauma. On the topic of self-blame in abuse victims, see N. Field et al., "Revictimization and Information Processing in Women Survivors of Childhood Sexual Abuse"; K. Ginzburg et al., "The Abuse-Related Beliefs Questionnaire for Survivors of Childhood Sexual Abuse"; and G. E. Wyatt, M. Newcomb, and S. M. Notgrass, "Internal and External Mediators of Women's Rape Experiences."

5. Much has been written about happiness and our individual predisposition

toward it. Two sources that do a good job covering the major points about this concept of happiness as a trait and about individual propensities toward subjective well-being are F. Fujita and E. Diener, "Life Satisfaction Set Point: Stability and Change"; and D. Watson, "Positive Affectivity: The Disposition to Experience Pleasurable Emotional States.

6. For a good explanation and review of the set-point theory of weight, see R. E. Keesey, "Physiological Regulation of Body Energy: Importance for Obesity."

7. It appears that even when dramatic things happen to us, good or bad, we tend to revert to our regular levels of happiness within a surprisingly short period of time, with certain exceptions. The following book provides a good review of the literature on how these changes make little difference, while providing some practical strategies to raise our happiness levels and keep them there: D. Lykken, *Happiness: What Studies on Twins Tell Us About Nature, Nurture, and the Happiness Set-Point.*

Chapter 6. Greater Than the Weight of Our Parts: Making Sense of It All

1. Aversion therapy is a type of therapy in which a negative experience is paired with the behavior you want to get rid of. For example, you give an alcoholic individual a drug that makes them very ill if they ingest an alcoholic beverage. Another word for aversion therapy is *counterconditioning.* So in that sense, the dumping reaction that the body has to the ingestion of certain foods or quantities of them after obesity surgery can act as an aversive experience that becomes paired with certain foods or quantities.

2. Typically, weight regain starts approximately eighteen to twenty-four months after surgery. Some researchers have attributed the weight gain to the disappearance of the dumping syndrome, others to coping difficulties, and yet others to the return of the binge-eating disorder that characterized a number of patients prior to surgery. Studies that have reported on and investigated this phenomenon include L. K. Hsu et al., "Nonsurgical Factors That Influence the Outcome of Bariatric Surgery: A Review"; P. S. Powers et al., "Eating Pathology Before and After Bariatric Surgery: A Prospective Study"; and H. J. Sugerman et al., "Gastric Bypass for Treating Severe Obesity.

3. In their study of twenty gastric bypass patients, "An Exploration of the Outcomes of Gastric Bypass Surgery for Morbid Obesity: Patient Characteristics and Indices of Success," C. R. Delin, J. M. Watts, and D. Bassett report that fear of confrontation and difficulty coping with life's demands were characteristic of patients who lost the least amount of weight.

Bibliography

Abell, S.C., and M.H.Richards. "The Relationship Between Body Shape Satisfaction and Self-esteem: An Investigation of Gender and Class Differences." *Journal of Youth and Adolescence* 25 (1996): 691–703.

Abramson, E.E., and S.Catalano. "Weight Loss and Sexual Behavior." *Journal of Obesity and Weight Reduction* 4 (1985): 268–73.

American Psychiatric Association Work Group on Eating Disorders. "Practice Guidelines for the Treatment of Patients With Eating Disorders (Revision)." *American Journal of Psychiatry* 157 (2000): 1–39.

Apple, R.F., J.Locke, and R.Peeples. *Preparing for Weight Loss Surgery: Therapist Guide.* New York: Oxford University Press, 2006.

———. New York: Oxford University Press, 2006. *Preparing for Weight Loss Surgery Workbook.*

Bachman, G., J.Bancroft, G.Braunstein, H.Burger, S.Davis, I.Dennerstein, I.Goldstein, et al. "Female Androgen Insufficiency: The Princeton Consensus Statement on Definition, Classification, and Assessment." *Fertility and Sterility* 77 (2002): 660–65.

Bandura, A. "Human Agency in Social Cognitive Theory." *American Psychologist* 44 (1989): 1175–84.

Bauchowitz, A.U., L.A.Gonder-Frederick, M.Olbrish, L.Azarbad, M.Ryee, M.Woodson, A.Miller, et al. "Psychosocial Evaluation of Bariatric Surgery Candidates: A Survey of Current Practices." *Psychosomatic Medicine* 67 (2005): 825–32.

Berg, F. *Health Risks of Obesity.* Hettinger, N.Dak.: Healthy Living Institute, 1993.

Bertakis, K.D., R.Azari, L.J.Helms, E.J.Callahan, and J.A.Robbins. "Gender Differences in the Utilization of Health Care Services." *Journal of Family Practice* 49 (2000): 147–52.

Bocchieri, L.E., M.Meana, and B.L.Fisher. "Perceived Psychosocial Outcomes of Gastric Bypass Surgery: A Qualitative Investigation." Paper presented at the annual meeting of the American Society for Bariatric Surgery, June 24–28, 2002, Las Vegas.

———. "Perceived Psychosocial Outcomes of Gastric Bypass Surgery: A Qualitative Study." *Obesity Surgery* 52 (2002): 155–65.

———. "The Question of Outcomes in Gastric Bypass Surgery." Poster presented at the annual convention of the Western Psychological Association, April 11–14, 2002, Irvine, Calif.

———. "Sexual Functioning Following Gastric Bypass Surgery: A Qualitative Investigation." Paper presented at the annual meeting of the Society for Sex Therapy and Research, March 14–17, 2002, Las Vegas.

Bocchieri-Ricciardi, L., M. Meana, B. Fisher, and R. Crosby. "Investigation of Weight-Related Relationship Adjustment in Female Obesity Surgery Patients." Paper presented at the annual meeting of the American Society for Bariatric Surgery, San Francisco, June 26–27, 2006.

Bowen, M. *Family Therapy in Clinical Practice.* Northvale, N.J.: Jason Aronson, 1978.

Brownell, K. D., and K. B. Horgen. *Food Fight.* New York: McGraw-Hill, 2004.

Burns, D. *The Feeling Good Handbook.* New York: Plume Publishing, 1999.

Camps, M. A., E. Zervos, S. Goode, and A. S. Rosemurgy. "Impact of Bariatric Surgery on Body Image Perception and Sexuality in Morbidly Obese Patients and Their Partners." *Obesity Surgery* 6 (1996): 356–60.

Canning, H., and J. Mayer. "Obesity: Its Possible Effect on College Acceptance." *New England Journal of Medicine* 275 (1966): 1172–74.

Cash, T., and E. A. Deagle. "The Nature and Extent of Body-Image Disturbances in Anorexia Nervosa and Bulimia Nervosa: A Meta-analysis." *International Journal of Eating Disorders* 22 (1997): 107–25.

Castelnuovo-Tedesco, P., J. Weinberg, D. Buchanan, and H. W. Scott. "Long-term Outcome of Jejuno-ileal Bypass Surgery for Superobesity: A Psychiatric Assessment." *American Journal of Psychiatry* 139 (1982): 1248–52.

Chamberlain, K. "Using Grounded Theory in Health Psychology: Practices, Premises, and Potential." In *Qualitative Health Psychology: Theories and Methods,* edited by M. Murray and K. Chamberlain, 183–201. Thousand Oaks, Calif.: Sage Publications, 1999.

Chandarana, P., R. Holliday, P. Conlon, and T. Deslippe. "Psychosocial Considerations in Gastric Stapling Surgery." *Journal of Psychosomatic Research* 32 (1988): 85–92.

Chen, E. Y., and M. Brown. "Obesity Stigma in Sexual Relationships." *Obesity Research* 13 (2005): 1393–97.

Counts, C. R., C. Jones, C. L. Frame, G. J. Jarvie, and C. C. Strauss. "The Perception of Obesity by Normal-Weight Versus Obese School-Age Children." *Child Psychiatry Human Development* 17 (1986): 113–20.

Cramer, P., and T. Steinwert. "Thin Is Good, Fat Is Bad: How Early Does It Begin?" *Journal of Applied Developmental Psychology* 19 (1998): 429–51.

Davis, M. M., K. Slish, C. Chao, and M. D. Cabana. "National Trends in Bariatric Surgery, 1996–2002." *Archives of Surgery* 141 (2006): 71–74.

Davis, S. R., S. L. Davison, S. Donath, and R. J. Bell. "Circulating Androgen Levels and Self-reported Sexual Function in Women." *Journal of the American Medical Association* 294 (2005): 91–96.

Delin, C. R., J. M. Watts, and D. I. Bassett. "An Exploration of the Outcomes of Gastric Bypass Surgery for Morbid Obesity: Patient Characteristics and Indices of Success." *Obesity Surgery* 5 (1995): 159–70.

Dubovsky, S. L., A. Haddenhorst, J. Murphy, R. D. Liechty, and D. A. Coyle. "A Preliminary Study of the Relationship Between Preoperative Depression and Weight Loss Following Surgery for Morbid Obesity." *International Journal of Psychiatry in Medicine* 15 (1985): 185–96.

Dymek, M. P., D. le Grange, K. Neven, and J. Alverdy. "Quality of Life After Gastric Bypass Surgery: A Cross-sectional Study." *Obesity Research* 10 (2002): 1135–42.

Ellis, B., and D. Symons. "Sex Differences in Sexual Fantasy: An Evolutionary Psychological Approach." *Journal of Sex Research* 27, no. 4 (1990): 527–55.

Else-Quest, N. M., J. S. Hyde, H. H. Goldsmith, and C. A. Van Hulle. "Gender Differences in Temperament: A Meta-analysis." *Psychological Bulletin* 132 (2006): 33–72.

Encinosa, W., D. Bernard, C. Steiner, and C. Chen. "Use and Costs of Bariatric Surgery and Prescription Weight-Loss Medications." *Health Affairs* 24 (2005): 1039–46.

Fairburn, C. G. *Overcoming Binge Eating.* New York: Guilford Press, 1995.

Fairburn, C. G., and K. D. Brownell, eds. *Eating Disorder and Obesity: A Comprehensive Handbook.* 2d ed. New York: Guilford Press, 2002.

Falkner, N. H., S. A. French, R. W. Jeffery, D. Neumark-Sztainer, N. E. Sherwood, and N. Morton. 1999. "Mistreatment Due to Weight: Prevalence and Sources of Perceived Mistreatment in Women and Men." *Obesity Research* 7 (1999): 572–76.

Field, N., C. C. Classen, L. D. Butler, C. Koopman, J. Zarcone, and D. Spiegel. "Revictimization and Information Processing in Women Survivors of Childhood Sexual Abuse." *Journal of Anxiety Disorders* 15 (2001): 459–69.

Fishbain, D. A., H. L. Rosomoff, R. B. Cutler, and R. S. Rosomoff. "Secondary Gain Concept: A Review of the Scientific Evidence." *Clinical Journal of Pain* 11 (1995): 6–21.

Fishbein, H. D. *Peer Prejudice and Discrimination: Evolutionary, Cultural, and Developmental Dynamics.* Boulder, Colo.: Westview Press, 1996.

Fishmann-Havstad, L., and A. R. Marston. "Weight Loss as an Aspect of Family Emotion and Process." *British Journal of Clinical Psychology* 23 (1984): 265–71.

Fredrickson, B., and T. Roberts. "Objectification Theory." *Psychology of Women Quarterly* 21 (1997): 173–206.

Fujita, F., and E. Diener. "Life Satisfaction Set Point: Stability and Change." *Journal of Personality and Social Psychology* 88 (2005): 158–64.

Furtado, M., and L. Schultz. *Recipes for Life After Weight-Loss Surgery: Delicious Dishes for Nourishing the New You.* Beverly, Mass.: Fair Winds Press, 2007.

Ganley, R. M. "Epistemology, Family Patterns, and Psychosomatics: The Case of Obesity." *Family Process* 25 (1986): 437–51.

Ginzburg, K., B. Arnow, S. Hart, W. Gardner, C. Koopman, C. C. Classen, J. Giese-Davis, et al. "The Abuse-Related Beliefs Questionnaire for Survivors of Childhood Sexual Abuse." *Child Abuse and Neglect* 30 (2006): 929–43.

Goble, L. K., C. S. W. Rand, and J. M. Kuldau. "Understanding Marital Relationships Following Obesity Surgery." *Family Therapy* 8 (1986): 196–202.

Goldberg, M. C., G. Cowan, and W. Y. Marcus. *Weight Loss Surgery: Is It Right for You?* New York: Square One Publishers, 2005.

Gould, J. C., M. J. Garren, V. Boll, and J. R. Starling. "Laparoscopic Gastric Bypass: Risk vs. Benefits up to Two Years Following Surgery in Super-Super Obese Patients." *Surgery* 140 (2006): 524–31.

Greenberger, D., and C. A. Padesky. *Mind Over Mood: Change How You Feel by Changing the Way You Think.* New York: Guilford Press, 1995.

Hafner, R. J. "Morbid Obesity: Effects on the Marital System of Weight Loss After Gastric Restriction." *Psychotherapy and Psychosomatics* 56 (1991): 162–66.

Harkaway, J. E. "Obesity: Reducing the Larger System." *Journal of Strategic and Systemic Therapies* 2 (1983): 2–16.

Hey, H., and U. Niebuhr-Jorgensen. "Jejuno-ileal Bypass Surgery in Obesity: Gynecological and Obstetrical Aspects." *Acta Obstetric Gynecologica Scandinavica* 60 (1981): 135–40.

Hoppe, R., and J. Ogden. "Practice Nurses' Beliefs About Obesity and Weight-Related Interventions in Primary Care." *International Journal of Obesity and Related Metabolic Disorders* 21 (1997): 141–46.

Hsu, L. K., P. N. Benotti, J. Dwyer, S. B. Roberts, E. Satzman, S. Shikora, B. J. Rolls, et al. "Nonsurgical Factors That Influence the Outcome of Bariatric Surgery: A Review." *Psychosomatic Medicine* 60 (1998): 338–46.

Janeway, J. M., K. J. Sparks, and R. S. Baker. *The Real Skinny on Weight Loss Surgery: An Indispensable Guide to What You Can Really Expect!* Onondaga, Mich.: Little Victories Press, 2005.

Keane, M. "Contemporary Beliefs About Mental Illness Among Medical Students:

Implications for Education and Practice." *Academic Psychiatry* 14 (1990): 172–77.

Keesey, R. E. "Physiological Regulation of Body Energy: Importance for Obesity." In *Obesity Theory and Therapy,* edited by A. J. Stunkard and T. A. Wadden, 77–96. 2d ed. New York: Raven Press, 1993.

Kendrick, M. L., and G. F. Dakin. "Surgical Approaches to Obesity." *Mayo Clinic Proceedings* 81 (2006): 18–24.

Keys, A., J. Brozek, A. Henschel, O. Mickelsen, and H. L. Taylor. *The Biology of Human Starvation.* 2 vols. Minneapolis: University of Minnesota Press, 1940.

Kinzl, J. F., E. Trefault, M. Fiala, A. Hotter, W. Biebl, and F. Aigner. "Partnership, Sexuality, and Sexual Disorders in Morbidly Obese Women: Consequence of Weight Loss After Gastric Banding." *Obesity Surgery* 11 (2001): 455–58.

Klein, D., J. Najman, A. F. Kohrman, and C. Munro. "Patient Characteristics That Elicit Negative Responses From Family Physicians." *Journal of Family Practice* 14 (1982): 881–88.

Kottke, T. E., R. N. Battista, G. H. DeFriese, and M. L. Brekke. "Attributes of Successful Smoking Cessation Interventions in Medical Practice: A Meta-analysis of 39 Controlled Trials." *Journal of the American Medical Association* 259 (1988): 2883–89.

Kurian, M. S., B. Thompson, and B. K. Davidson. *Weight Loss Surgery for Dummies.* New York: Wiley, 2005.

Laumann, E. O., J. H. Gagnon, R. T. Michael, and S. Michaels. *The Social Organization of Sexuality: Sexual Practices in the United States.* Chicago: University of Chicago Press, 1994.

Levine, P., M. Bontmpo-Saray, W. B. Inabnet, and M. Urban-Skuros. *Eating Well After Weight Loss Surgery: Over 140 Delicious Low-Fat, High-Protein Recipes to Enjoy in the Weeks, Months, and Years After Surgery.* New York: Marlowe, 2004.

Lykken, D. *Happiness: What Studies on Twins Show Us About Nature, Nurture, and the Happiness Set-Point.* New York: Golden Books, 1999.

MacLean, L. D., B. M. Rhode, and C. W. Nohr. "Late Outcomes of Isolated Gastric Bypass." *Annals of Surgery* 231 (2000): 524–28.

Markus, H. "Self-Schemata and Processing Information About the Self." *Journal of Personality and Social Psychology* 35 (1977): 63–78.

Markus, H., R. Hamill, and K. P. Sentis. 1987. "Thinking Fat: Self Schemas for Body Weight and the Processing of Weight-Relevant Information." *Journal of Applied Social Psychology* 17 (1987): 50–71.

Marshall, J. R., and J. Neill. "The Removal of a Psychosomatic Symptom: Effects on the Marriage." *Family Process* 16 (1977): 273–80.

Martin, P. R., and N. Petry. "Are Non-Substance-Related Addictions Really Addictions?" *American Journal on Addictions* 14 (2005): 1–7.

McArthur, L., and J. Ross. "Attitudes of Registered Dietitians Toward Personal Overweight and Overweight Clients." *Journal of the American Dietetic Association* 97 (1997): 63–66.

McKenna J. W., and K. N. Williams. "Crafting Effective Tobacco Counter-Advertisements: Lessons From a Failed Campaign Directed at Teenagers." *Public Health Reports* 108 (1993): 85–89.

McTiernan, A., L. Wu, C. Chen, R. Chlebowski, Y. Mossavar-Rahmani, F. Modugno, M. G. Perri, et al. "Relation of BMI and Physical Activity to Sex Hormones in Post-menopausal Women." *Obesity* 14 (2006): 1662–77.

Mitchell, J. E., and M. de Zwaan, eds. *Bariatric Surgery: Psychosocial Assessment and Treatment.* New York: Brunner/Mazel, 2005.

Neill, J. R., J. R. Marshall, and C. E. Yale. "Marital Changes After Intestinal Bypass Surgery." *Journal of the American Medical Association* 240 (1978): 447–50.

Nguyen, N. T., J. Root, K. Zainabadi, A. Sabio, S. Chalifoux, C. M. Stevens, S. Mavandadi, et al. "Accelerated Growth of Bariatric Surgery With the Introduction of Minimally Invasive Surgery." *Archives of Surgery* 140 (2005): 1198–1202.

Ogden, C. L., C. D. Fryar, M. D. Carroll, and K. M. Flegal. "Mean Body Weight, Height, and Body Mass Index, United States, 1960–2002." In *Advance Data From Vital and Health Statistics.* No. 347. Hyattsville, Md.: National Center for Health Statistics, 2004.

Oliak, D., G. H. Ballantyne, R. J. Davies, A. Wasielewski, and H. J. Schmidt. "Short-term Results of Laparoscopic Gastric Bypass in Patients With BMI >60." *Obesity Surgery* 12 (2003): 643–47.

Overmeier, J. B., and M. E. P. Seligman. "Effects of Inescapable Shock Upon Subsequent Escape and Avoidance Responding." *Journal of Comparative and Physiological Psychology* 63 (1967): 28–33.

Petersen, C., S. F. Maier, and M. E. P. Seligman. *Learned Helplessness: A Theory for the Age of Personal Control.* New York: Oxford University Press, 1995.

Plomin, R., J. C. DeFries, G. E. McClearn, and M. Rutter. *Behavioral Genetics.* New York: Freeman, 1997.

Pories, W. J., and G. M. Pratt. "Commentary: Quality Control of Bariatric Surgery." *Bariatric Nursing and Surgical Patient Care* 1 (2006): 53–59.

Porter, L. C., and R. S. Wampler. "Adjustment to Rapid Weight Loss." *Families, Systems, and Health* 18 (2000): 35–54.

Powers, P. S., A. Perez, F. Boyd, and A. Rosemurgy. "Eating Pathology Before and After Bariatric Surgery: A Prospective Study." *International Journal of Eating Disorders* 25 (1997): 293–300.

Prochaska, J. O., and W. F. Velicer. "The Transtheoretical Model of Health Behavior Change." *American Journal of Health Promotion* 12 (1997): 38–48.

Puhl R., and K. D. Brownell. "Bias, Discrimination, and Obesity." *Obesity Research* 9 (2005): 788–805.

Rand, C. S. W., K. Kowalske, and J. M. Kuldau. "Characteristics of Marital Improvement Following Obesity Surgery." *Psychosomatics* 25 (1984): 221–26.

Rand, C. S. W., J. M. Kuldau, and L. Robbins. "Surgery for Obesity and Marriage Quality." *Journal of the American Medical Association* 247 (1982): 1419–22.

Resnick, M. D. "Protective Factors, Resiliency, and Healthy Youth Development." *Adolescent Medicine: State of the Art Reviews* 11 (2000): 157–64.

Richardson, S. A., N. Goodman, A. H. Hastorf, and S. M. Dornbusch. "Cultural Uniformity in Reaction to Physical Disabilities." *American Sociological Review* 26 (1961): 241–47.

Rimer, B. K. "Understanding the Acceptance of Mammography by Women." *Annals of Behavioral Medicine* 14 (1992): 197–203.

Roberts, B. W., and W. F. DelVecchio. "The Rank-Order Consistency of Personality Traits From Childhood to Old-Age: A Quantitative Review of Longitudinal Studies." *Psychological Bulletin* 126 (2000): 3–25.

Roehling, M. V. "Weight-Based Discrimination in Employment: Psychological and Legal Aspects." *Personnel Psychology* 52 (1999): 969–1017.

Rosenfield, S., M. C. Lennon, and H. R. White. "The Self and Mental Health: Self-salience and the Emergence of Internalizing and Externalizing Problems." *Journal of Health and Social Behavior* 46 (2005): 323–40.

Saris, H. M. Wim. "Very Low-Calorie Diets and Sustained Weight Loss." *Obesity Research* 9 (2001): S295–S301.

Schiavi, R. C., D. White, J. Mandeli, and A. C. Levine. "Effect of Testosterone Administration on Sexual Behavior and Mood in Men With Erectile Dysfunction." *Archives of Sexual Behavior* 26 (1997): 231–41.

Serdula, M. K., A. H. Mokdad, D. F. Williamson, D. A. Galuska, and G. W. Heath. "Prevalence of Attempting Weight Loss and Strategies for Controlling Weight." *Journal of the American Medical Association* 282 (1999): 1353–58.

Shifren, J. L., G. D. Braunstein, J. A. Simon, P. R. Casson, J. E. Buster, G. P. Redmond, R. E. Burki, et al. "Transdermal Testosterone Treatment in Women With Impaired Sexual Function After Oopherectomy." *New England Journal of Medicine* 343 (2000): 682–88.

Skrzypek, S., P. M. Wehmeier, and H. Remschmidt. "Body Image Assessment Using Body Size Estimation in Recent Studies on Anorexia Nervosa: A Brief Review." *European Child and Adolescent Psychiatry* 10 (2001): 215–21.

Spitzer, R. L., S. Yanovski, T. Wadden, R. Wing, M. D. Marcus, A. Stunkard, M. Devlin, et al. "Binge-Eating Disorder: Its Further Validation in a Multisite Study." *International Journal of Eating Disorders* 13 (1993): 137–53.

Staffieri, J. R. "A Study of Social Stereotype of Body Image in Children." *Journal of Personality and Social Psychology* 7 (1961): 101–4.

Stice, E. "Risk and Maintenance Factors for Eating Pathology: A Meta-analytic Review." *Psychological Bulletin* 128 (2002): 825–48.

Stuart, R. B., and B. Jacobson. *Weight, Sex, and Marriage: A Delicate Balance.* New York: Norton, 1989.

Stunkard, A. J. "Current Views of Obesity." *American Journal of Medicine* 100 (1996): 230–36.

Stunkard, A. J., and T. I. Sorenson. "Obesity and Socioeconomic Status: A Complex Relation." *New England Journal of Medicine* 329 (1993): 1036–37.

Sugerman, H. J., J. M. Kellum, K. M. Engle, L. Wolfe, J. V. Starkey, R. Birkenhauer, P. Fletcher, et al. "Gastric Bypass for Treating Severe Obesity." *American Journal of Clinical Nutrition* 55 (1992): 560–66.

Sugerman, H. J., G. L. Londrey, J. M. Kellum, L. Wold, T. Liszka, K. M. Engle, R. Birkenhauer, et al. "Weight Loss With Vertical Banded Gastroplasty and Roux-Y Gastric Bypass for Morbid Obesity With Selective Versus Random Assignment." *American Journal of Surgery* 157 (1989): 93–102.

Technology Assessment Conference Statement. "Methods for Voluntary Weight Loss and Control." *Annals of Internal Medicine* 119 (1993): 764–70.

Thirlby, R. C., and J. Randall. "A Genetic 'Obesity Risk Index' for Patients With Morbid Obesity." *Obesity Surgery* 12 (2002): 25–29.

Tiggeman, M. "Body-Size Dissatisfaction: Individual Differences in Age and Gender and Relationship With Self-esteem." *Personality and Individual Differences* 13 (1992): 39–43.

Wadden, T. A., and D. B. Sarwer. "Behavioral Assessment of Candidates for Bariatric Surgery: A Patient-Oriented Approach." *Obesity* 14 (2006): S53–S62.

Watson, D. "Positive Affectivity: The Disposition to Experience Pleasurable Emotional States." In *Handbook of Positive Psychology,* edited by C. R. Snyder and S. Lopez, 106–19. New York: Oxford University Press, 2002.

Weiderman, M. W. "Extramarital Sex: Prevalence and Correlates in a National Survey." *Journal of Sex Research* 34 (1997): 167–74.

Woodward, B. G. *A Complete Guide to Obesity Surgery: Everything You Need to Know About Weight Loss Surgery and How to Succeed.* Victoria, B.C.: Trafford, 2001.

Wyatt, G. E., M. Newcomb, and S. M. Notgrass. "Internal and External Mediators of Women's Rape Experiences." In *Rape and Sexual Assault,* edited by A. Wolpert Burgess, 32–43. New York: Garland, 1991.

Index

Abell, S. C., 246n2

achievement, 71–72, 141–42

addiction: to food, 25–26, 153, 246n16; obese thinking as, 153

American Obesity Association, 235, 243n1

American Society for Metabolic and Bariatric Surgery, 3, 239, 241n3

American Society of Bariatric Physicians, 238–39

anger, 76, 86–87, 103. *See also* revenge

assertiveness: 12, 230; with family of origin, 127; in friendships, 122–24

attention: decrease in, 199–200; negative reactions to, 82–84; positive reactions to, 84; romantic, 73–80, 143

attributions: for change, 144–47; for failure, 166–72, 175–80. See also responsibility

Bachman, G., 251n15

Bandura, A., 249n8

Bassett, D., 254n3

Berg, F., 243n1

Bertakis, K. D., 242n9

binge eating, 12, 154, 162–63, 253n2. *See also* emotional eating

body image: and self-esteem, 62–63, 246n2; in eating disorders, 154, 252–53n6; in obesity, 22–23, 154

Brownell, K. D., 247n3

Burns, D., 246n18

Canning, H., 244n6

Cash, T., 252n6

Centers for Disease Control and Prevention, 235–36, 241n2

Chamberlain, K., 243n11

children: impact of obesity on, 110–11, 113; and support of parents, 113. *See also* parenting

communication, 223–24, 230–31

Counts, C. R., 243–44n4

Cramer, P., 243–44n4

Dakin, G. F., 253n1

Davidson, B. K., 242n6

Davis, S. R., 251n15

Deagle, E. A., 252n6

death: fear of, 29–33; obesity-related causes of, 11, 243n1; rate from surgery, 2, 241n1

defeatism, 19, 139, 152, 174–75

Delin, C. R., 254n3

denial, 20–22, 177